Fertility
Diet

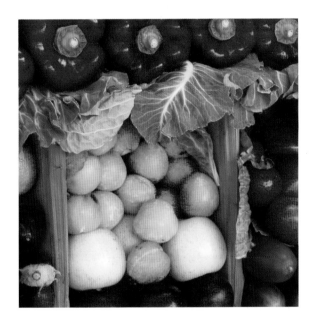

Tasha Jennings ND

Tasha Jennings holds degrees in naturopathy, nutrition and herbal medicine and has over 10 years' experience in the field. She has extensive experience in clinical practice and is also an expert writer, trainer and presenter. She is a regular keynote speaker at medical and health conferences and also runs trainings and seminars for medical and other health care professionals. She is an active and ongoing contributor to major media publications including newspapers, magazines, medical journals and websites. Continually inspired by innovative research in her field, Tasha progressed into product and program development and has been instrumental in the development of prominent vitamin and supplement ranges as well as a successful pharmaceutical health and weight loss program. Combining her clinical and business skills, she recently established her own company Zycia, meaning 'life'. Zycia specialises in pre and postnatal nutrition to support life in its earliest stages and help provide optimal outcomes for mother and baby (www.zycia.com.au).
Tasha is now a new Mum herself and enjoys using her knowledge to inspire others to live healthier, happier lives.

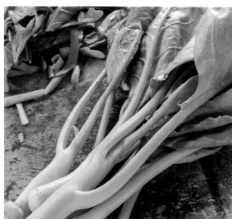

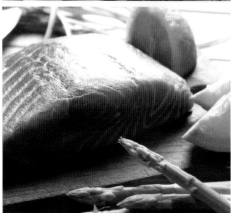

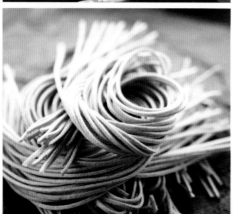

Published by:
Wilkinson Publishing Pty Ltd
ACN 006 042 173
Level 4, 2 Collins St Melbourne, Victoria, Australia 3000
Ph: +61 3 9654 5446
www.wilkinsonpublishing.com.au

International distribution by Pineapple Media Limited
(www.pineapple-media.com) ISSN 2200-0135

Creator: Jennings, Tasha, author.

Title: Fertility diet / Tasha Jennings N.D.

ISBN: 9781922178992 (paperback)

Subjects: Fertility, Human—Nutritional aspects.
                Human reproduction—Nutritional aspects.
                Woman—Health and hygiene.
                Cooking (Natural foods).
                Diet.

Dewey Number: 612.6

Layout Design: Corinda Cook, Tango Media Pty Ltd

Cover Design: Alicia Freile, Tango Media Pty Ltd

Photos by agreement with Thinkstock/iStock.

Contents

The Fertility Guide

Most of us take our fertility for granted. We assume that when we decide that we're ready to start a family we'll simply stop using contraception, fall pregnant within a few weeks and soon have a growing belly, food cravings and a baby on the way.

If only it were really that simple. The fact is that even the healthiest couples have only a 20 to 25 per cent chance of achieving a successful pregnancy each month, while 1 in 8 couples will experience conception difficulties – with this figure expected to double in the next decade.

So what can you do to boost your fertility and maximise your chances of getting pregnant?

That's where this book comes in, providing all the facts and information to allow you to manage and enhance your own fertility and make informed decisions about your reproductive health.

"You may encounter many defeats, but you must not be defeated. In fact, it my be necessary to encounter the defeats so you can know who you are, what you can rise from and how you can still come out of it"

– Maya Angelou

My Story

My reason for specialising in fertility and conception was initially a very personal one. As a very fit, healthy 30 year old I saw no reason why I wouldn't conceive as soon as we decided we were ready. However 12 months down the track I realised it was not going to be that easy.

My menstrual cycle had been a little irregular but nothing too extreme. Most months my period would just come and go, no symptoms or pain, so I saw no reason that there was anything amiss. I'd never charted my cycle, even when we were 'trying' during those first 12 months. In hindsight I'd been pretty casual about the whole process. I knew I should ovulate around mid-cycle so as long as we were trying around that time we should be fine, right? Unfortunately not.

At this point I began charting my cycle using the temperature charting method outlined in this book. For the first month I had barely any change in temperature at all. So I charted it again the second month, then the third, all with the same result. I was quite astonished, and as someone who probably should know better, I was a little embarrassed that I didn't realise I wasn't ovulating at all.

Being a Naturopath and Nutritionist I was keen to support my body with the best nutrition possible so I also began researching the latest nutritional information to help me ovulate, boost my fertility and prepare my body for pregnancy. Amazed at the fascinating new research I was discovering, what started our as a small personal journey became a large-scale project as I met and spoke with nutritional researchers from all over the globe.

At the same time we made an appointment to see a fertility specialist/obstetrician who ran tests for both of us, confirming that I wasn't ovulating but thankfully that I was otherwise healthy, as was my husband.

During the wait to see my fertility specialist I had already commenced my own supportive treatment of herbs and nutrients. This, combined with the pre-scribed medication from my specialist, enabled me to conceive the very first month!

After a wonderful, healthy pregnancy and natural birth, I am very pleased to say I have a thriving 2 year old son and a little sister due in less than 4 weeks!

Although my conception journey was relatively short compared to many couples I speak with, the 18 months we were trying, felt like years. So can empathise with any couples struggling with fertility issues.

I believe I am like many women, who feel assured that their ability to have children will always be there whenever they are ready. Having been very career focused during my twenties, children were not on my radar at all. Yet I always knew I wanted to have family, I just felt certain that it would happen when I was ready.

As many women do, I then blamed myself for not being able to easily conceive. Maybe if I hadn't been so focused on my career or so stressed, maybe if I had have done this or that, everything would be fine. So I'd like to pass this on to all women and couples trying to start their family. The blame game does not help. The past is the past, what's done is done. Focus on the future and you can take control of your fertility.

I highly recommend the assistance of a fertility specialist. The world of reproductive technology has made amazing breakthroughs. I feel privileged to live in an era where couples who

may have otherwise been infertile, now have the chance to have the family they always dreamed of. However I also strongly recommend the use of natural dietary and lifestyle changes to improve your chances of conception, either alone or alongside any medical assistance that might be required.

As outlined in this book, there are many lifestyle and dietary changes you can make that will significantly increase your chances of conception. Even if you are you are commencing IVF treatment, you know your body better than anyone and you have more invested in this journey than anyone. You can help improve the quality of your eggs, you can help support regular ovulation, you can support the health your uterus, you can improve your overall reproductive health and your partners to help make any medical inter-vention required all the most successful.

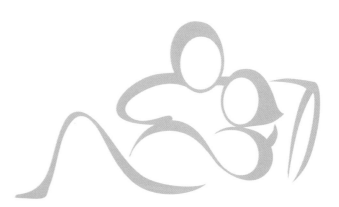

The basics

MENSTRUAL CYCLE

The 'normal' cycle - How it works

The menstrual cycle is an amazing and complex series of events all primarily aimed at ensuring a healthy environment for reproduction. This cycle helps keep the uterine conditions ideal for implantation by regularly shedding the uterine lining (endometrium) each month. An average menstrual cycle lasts 28 days, yet it's believed that only around 20 percent of women have an 'average' cycle. In reality the cycle can last anywhere between 21 and 35 days.

The menstrual cycle is regulated by two major hormones - follicle stimulating hormone (FSH) and luteinising hormone (LH). The balance of these hormones stimulates ovulation and promotes the production of either progesterone or estrogen in the ovaries.

THE CYCLE HAS THREE MAJOR PHASES:

Phase 1 – Follicular Phase
Phase 2 – Ovulatory Phase
Phase 3 – Luteal Phase

The Follicular Phase

The first half of your cycle is called the follicular. This phase begins on the first day of the menstrual bleed. At the beginning of this phase both estrogen and progesterone levels are low, causing the tops layers of the endometrium to shed, forming the menstrual bleed. During this time FSH begins to rise, stimulating the growth of between 3 to 30 follicles within the ovaries, each follicle housing an egg. While the follicles are developing they produce increasing levels of estrogen, which stimulates the thickening of the endometrium in preparation for potential implantation of a fertilised egg. The level of FSH decreases slightly before ovulation and only one of the developing follicles will remain and continue to develop a mature egg. This is known as the dominant follicle (in rare cases, 2 or more eggs will mature, which can result in multiple birth). Estrogen levels continue to rise during the follicular phase until reaching a peak just before ovulation. The average follicular phase lasts around 13 – 14 days. However this phase is the most likely to vary significantly in length.

The Ovulatory Phase

The peak in estrogen just before ovulation, triggers a surge in LH and, to a lesser extent, another rise in FSH. The sharp rise in LH triggers the follicle to rupture and release the egg (or in rare cases multiple eggs) from the ovary. As soon as the egg has been released at ovulation, FSH and LH levels sharply decline. If fertilisation doesn't occur, the egg will degenerate in the uterus about 12 – 24 hours after its release from the ovary and will then be shed during the next menstrual bleed. The average ovulatory phase lasts around 16 – 32 hours, beginning with the surge in LH and ending when the egg is released. (Read more about ovulation and how it impacts fertility on page 10 'All about ovulation')

The Luteal Phase

The follicle in which the egg grew then closes and forms the corpus luteum.

Stimulated by the influence of LH, the corpus luteum releases increasing amounts of progesterone. Progesterone further prepares the thickened endometrium for implantation by supporting the development of glandular structures and blood vessels that would nourish a developing embryo. Estrogen levels decrease slightly as progesterone levels increase to become the dominant hormone during this phase. If an egg is not fertilised, the corpus luteum regresses after around 14 days. This signals a drop in estrogen and progesterone, which stimulates the shedding of the endometrium and the beginning of a new cycle.

If an egg is fertilised and implanted, the cells around the embryo secrete human chorionic gonadotropin hormone. This hormone maintains the activity of the corpus luteum, which continues to release progesterone until the foetus can take over its own hormone production. It is this hormone that pregnancy tests detect to indicate a positive pregnancy test.

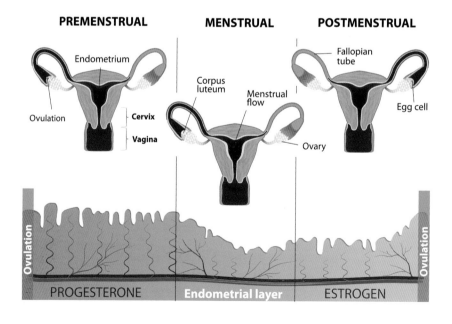

HOW DOES REPRODUCTION HAPPEN?

Women are born with around 1 million potential eggs (or follicles), which decrease to around 300,000 – 400,000 by the time menstruation commences. Each month one dominant egg (or in rarer cases multiple eggs) is released from the ovary to begin its journey into one of the fallopian tubes where tiny hair like cilia, sweep the egg towards the uterus.

During sexual intercourse around 200 million sperm are released at a rate of up to 45km (28 miles) per hour! This rapid speed slows to around 30cm per hour as they race towards the egg. In the average male around 15 – 45 million of these will be healthy enough to fertilise an egg, however only around 400 will survive after ejaculation. Of these 400 hundred surviving sperm, about 40 will be strong enough to reach the fallopian tube and the vicinity of the egg. These remaining 40 sperm then go through a process called capacitation, which is an explosion enabling the sperm to penetrate the outer layer of the egg. After this process only one, if any, sperm will remain to fertilise the egg. Fertilisation most commonly occurs in the fallopian tube.

When a sperm reaches and penetrates an egg, it will claim it as its own, by altering the surface of the egg to prevent other sperm from entering. The gender of the child as well as their physical characteristics including facial features, hair, eye and skin colour and to a certain extent their personality traits, the way they think, feel, act, respond and basically everything that makes them 'them', are determined at this moment as 46 chromosomes (23 from the mother and 23 from the father) combine together to commence the beginning of a new life.

A fertilised egg is known as a zygote. The zygote generally reaches the uterus within 3 – 5 days of being fertilised, during which time it has already begun to divide and grow. Once in the uterus, the zygote continues to divide and grow where it becomes a blastocyst. The blastocyst then attaches and implants into the endometrium about 5 – 8 days after fertilisation. This whole process is complete within 9 – 10 days.

After implantation, the inner cells of the blastocyst will divide into what will become the embryo and the outer cells will nestle into the endometrium to become the placenta. The placental cells will then develop further to form an outer layer of membranes known as the chorion, which encase and protect the blastocyst as well as an inner layer, known as the amnion, which forms the amniotic sac. The amniotic sac is fully formed by around 10 – 12 days after fertilisation. This sac will then fill with amniotic fluid and expand to house the developing embryo. The amniotic sac will be your baby's first home where it will continue to develop for the entire pregnancy.

In ideal conditions, this process runs very smoothly. However in reality, around half of all fertilised eggs fail to develop.

The initial development of an embryo proceeds very rapidly. Only 4 weeks after fertilisation, the neural tube - which connects the brain and spinal cord - has already developed and closed. This process relies on essential dietary nutrients including folate and choline for healthy growth, without which, neural tube defects may occur. Just 10 weeks after fertilisation almost all organs are completely formed. It is during these critical 10 weeks that the embryo is most vulnerable to birth defects and miscarriage.

In this book we outline how you can help improve your chances not only of fertilisation but a successful implantation and the healthy growth and development of your precious baby.

ALL ABOUT OVULATION

How it works

Ovulation is the process by which an egg is released from your ovary, where it then flows into your fallopian tube and is pushed towards your uterus (womb). About 3 – 30 eggs begin to develop within the follicles in your ovaries each month until one takes over as the 'dominant' follicle and will produce a fully mature egg. In rarer cases, more than one follicle will produce a fully mature egg, and this can result in twin or multiple birth. The remaining eggs will simply degenerate in a process called atresia. There appears to be no pattern as to which of your two ovaries produces the dominant follicle and releases the egg each month.

It is during the eggs journey through the fallopian tube that fertilisation can occur if sperm are present. Once released from the ovary an egg will be viable for only 12 – 24 hours. For conception to occur, sperm must be present during this window.

Ovulation generally occurs between day 10 and day 19 of your cycle. Knowing the exact timing of your ovulatory phase greatly increases your chances of conception. Sperm can survive within the female reproductive system for 2 – 5 days. Therefore having sex 3 – 4 days prior to and up to 24 hours after ovulation maximises your chances of conception.

How to know when/ if you're ovulating

These techniques are designed not only to check when, but also if you are ovulating. It's important to remember that menstruation can occur without ovulation and, although less common, ovulation can occur without the presence of a menstrual cycle.

Temperature charting

The hormonal changes that occur during the menstrual cycle influence our Basal Body Temperature (BBT). By charting your temperature each morning you will begin to establish a pattern that reflects your individual changes. These changes indicate when and if ovulation is occurring. Temperature does not predict when ovulation will happen, because temperature changes occur after ovulation has occurred, however charting your temperature each month will help to establish your unique pattern enabling you to better predict your likely fertile days each month.

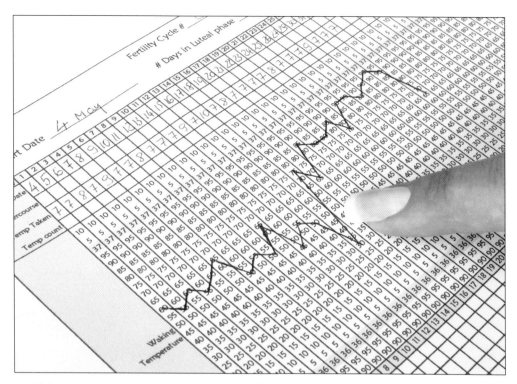

Using a digital or mercury oral thermometer, you need to take your temperature via mouth (or vaginally, however whichever method you use, you must stick with this method as vaginal temperature is slightly higher than oral temperature) at the same time each morning before you get out of bed. For the reading to be most accurate you must not eat, drink (or hopefully you're not smoking!) and have had at least 3 hours sleep before you take your temperature. The exact temperature is less important than the change in temperature.

Anywhere between 96 – 98 degrees Fahrenheit or 35.5 – 36.5 degrees Celsius is normal before ovulation and anywhere between 97 – 99 degrees Fahrenheit or 36.2 – 37.2 degrees Celsius is normal after ovulation. When you ovulate your temperature will rise and remain higher for at least 10 days before dropping back to the starting temperature ready for the next menstrual cycle to commence. If your temperature spikes but remains high for less than 10 days, this can indicate that ovulation has occurred however your luteal phase is too short to establish a pregnancy.

Your most fertile days fall 2-3 days before temperature reaches its peak and for about 1 day after. You should also notice a slight drop in temperature before the rise. This drop can help you predict that ovulation is about to occur, indicating that you are commencing your fertile period.

When charting your temperature it's important to be mindful that other external factors, aside from hormones, can influence basal temperature.

THESE INCLUDE:
✓ Being unwell
✓ High stress levels
✓ Shift work
✓ Interrupted sleep

Mucus testing

Another technique you can use to help predict your fertile days is to monitor your cervical mucus. The natural mucus we secrete changes colour and consistency during your cycle. These changes are influenced by the hormonal changes occurring during your cycle and play a role in either hindering or supporting the progression of sperm to the uterus. Some women secrete more mucus than others and some women secrete very little at all. The amount is less important than the colour and consistency.

As your estrogen levels rise towards ovulation, you will notice that your mucus becomes a thinner, clearer consistency. It also becomes quite slippery and stretchy, much like the consistency and colour of egg white. This is your fertile mucus, acting like a slippery dip, to speed the sperms journey through the cervix and uterus and into the fallopian tube where it can finally reach its destination, your egg. Studies show that the last day of your 'slippery' mucus, is your peak day of fertility as ovulation generally occurs within a day of your peak day. Your peak fertile day may also be associated with physical symptoms such as a feeling of fullness, softness or gentle swelling in the vaginal area. To optimise your chances of conception it's ideal to be having sex in the days leading up to the peak as well as on the peak day and potentially the day after your peak. Most women will start to recognise the peak firstly by the definite change in mucus secretions the next day, from slippery to more dry and sticky, possibly damp.

Cervical Position

As with your cervical mucus, the position of your cervix naturally changes throughout your cycle to either encourage or help block sperm entering the fallopian tubes to reach the egg. You will also notice changes in the feel and texture of your uterus as you progress through the different stages of your cycle.

Performing a self-examination can take some practice. It's best done after a shower or even during a bath. Find a position that is comfortable for you and use this same position each time so you're drawing the same comparisons each time. Gently insert one or two fingers into the entrance of your vagina and feel for the cervix, which is located towards the upper front. By doing this regularly you will start to notice the unique changes corresponding to the timing in your cycle.

The menstrual bleeding phase
The cervix will be positioned quite low during the bleeding phase of your cycle. You should be able to reach it easily and will notice that it may feel open, kind of like your ear or nose. This position allows blood to easily flow out. It will also feel quite firm during this phase

When bleeding stops
When you come to the end of your period your cervix will still be positioned low down and feel firm but it will now be closed.

Leading up to ovulation
As your body prepares for the egg to be released at ovulation, your cervix will move higher up. You will also notice that it becomes softer and moister.

At ovulation

At the height of your ovulation phase, just as your egg is being released, your cervix is in the optimum position for conception. It will feel very soft, moist and open, more like your mouth and lips than your ear or nose during this phase. It will now be positioned quite high, you may not even be able to feel it because it's either out of reach or the softness may blend in with the vagina walls. This is the ideal position to support the journey of sperm to the egg. Now is the time to be having sex!

After ovulation

Once ovulation occurs, the cervix will begin to lower down and become firmer again. The cervix will now close tightly. This may happen immediately after ovulation or may take up to a few days.

If pregnancy occurs

If an egg is fertilised and implanted into the uterus, the cervix will rise back up and become soft again. However this time it will remain tightly closed.

If pregnancy doesn't occur

The uterus will remain closed and firm until the next menstrual period is due to begin

Ovulation test kits

Ovulation test kits are another way to help pin point your fertile window.

THESE COME IN THE FORM OF:

✓ Urine based test kits
✓ Salivary based test kits

Urine based test kits

These kits work by measuring the level of luteinising hormone (LH) in urine. There is always a small amount of LH present in blood and urine, however the volume of LH increases 2 to 5-fold 1 to 2 days prior to ovulation to stimulate release of the egg. Measuring when this surge is occurring provides an indication that ovulation is about to occur. The 3 days immediately after commencement of the LH surge is the window during which you are most likely to conceive.

When using urine-based kits it is best to follow the directions outlined on the packed as these can vary slightly between brands. However, in general it's best, although not essential, to test your urine at around the same time each day and ideally not first thing in the morning as this may miss the first day of your LH surge. Around 2 – 2:30pm appears to be ideal timing.

"Making a decision to have a child is momentous. It's to decide forever to have your heart go walking outside your body."

~ Elizabeth Stone

Also avoid drinking too much liquid prior to the test as this may dilute urine. Read the results within 10 minutes of performing the test. Positive tests won't disappear however a false positive may register after 10 minutes. Therefore once the results have been read, the test should be thrown out.

Urine based ovulation kits are around 99% accurate, making them one of the most reliable measures of ovulation, however they are not fool proof. It is possible for LH to surge without ovulation occurring. You may also experience false LH surges prior to the actual surge. However their strong reliability still makes them one of the best methods for predicting ovulation at home.

Salivary-based test kits

Using a tiny microscope, these kits enable you to visualise the changes in saliva patterns, stimulated by a change in hormone levels. Estrogen increases the salt content of your saliva. When this salt dries, if forms a fern-like pattern which can be seen through the microscope. This fern-like pattern indicates the presence of a high level of estrogen, which is most likely to occur in the few days leading up to ovulation. So when you see this pattern, the 3 – 4 days following this will be your most fertile.

Saliva based test kits aren't quite as accurate as urine based test kits. This is due to the fact that the fern-like patter may be present at other times during your cycle depending on your hormone levels. For some people, it may also be hard to accurately identify the fern-like pattern through the microscope. However, this type of kit can be a more popular option due to the convenience of testing as well as the ability to use the same test over and over for around 2 years.

Fertility medications can impact the accuracy of both kits, so best to speak with your specialist if you are taking any prescribed hormonal medication.

YOUR UTERUS

The uterus (or womb as it is commonly known) is quite simply an amazing organ. It is our baby's first home. A place in which a tiny fertilised egg (zygote) has the opportunity to develop into a healthy, thriving human being.

A normal uterus is a hollow muscular organ about the size and shape of a pear but has the ability to expand and stretch considerably to accommodate a growing foetus. In its non-pregnant state the uterus can hold around a teaspoon of liquid. During pregnancy it can expand up to 500 times its normal size!

The uterus is made up of 3 layers, the perimetrium (the thin outer layer), the myometrium, (the strong muscular layer in the middle) and the endometrium that forms the uterine lining. The uterus is extremely strong. In fact the uterine muscle (myometrium) is one of the strongest muscles in the body enabling the strong, rhythmic contractions required for child-birth and to a lesser extent, to expel the endometrial lining each month.

The uterus is constantly renewing its lining to prepare for impending implantation of a fertilised egg. This can be seen in the monthly shedding of the uterine lining, which occurs each month. In fact the sole purpose of the menstrual cycle is to prepare the uterus for pregnancy. The endometrium, or uterine lining, is made up of 2 layers, which merge together to appear as one. However they perform very different roles. The basal layer remains intact as a constant cover for the myometrium (uterine muscle). The basal layer changes very little in response to the hormonal fluctuations during menstruation and is not shed during the period. The functional layer on the other hand responds greatly to the monthly changes in hormonal activity and is shed as menstrual blood and rebuilt each month.

Anatomy

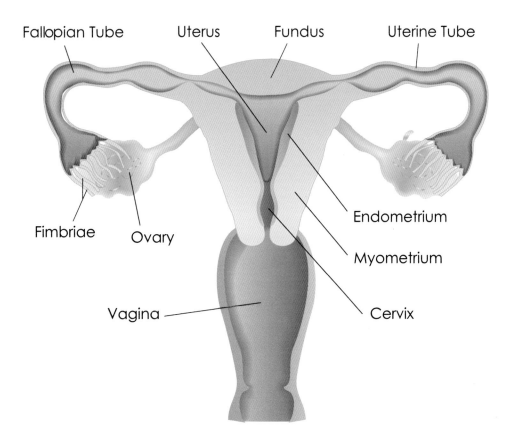

Fallopian Tube   Uterus   Fundus   Uterine Tube

Fimbriae   Ovary

Endometrium

Myometrium

Vagina

Cervix

What affects fertility? Men and women

AGE MATTERS

Women

Age is the most important determinant of your fertility. Up to the age of 35, couples have approximately 20 – 25% chance of conceiving each month. Fertility declines markedly after the age of 35, reducing by approximately 50% at age 40 and continues to drop before ceasing at menopause.

> THE SIGNIFICANT DECLINE IN FERTILITY IS DUE TO:
> ✓ reduced egg quality and quantity
> ✓ lowered estrogen levels
> ✓ increased follicle stimulating hormone (FSH), produced in response to the lack of responsiveness in the ovaries
> ✓ less frequent ovulation
> ✓ reduced cervical mucus
> ✓ reduced blood flow to the reproductive organs

Women over 40 are also more likely to suffer miscarriage due to high chromosomal abnormalities relating to the reduced egg quality.

Although assisted reproduction techniques have come a long way in the past decade, IVF is not the magic bullet many people would like to believe. In fact, women aged 40 – 42 have a significantly reduced success rate if less than 5 viable eggs are produced and most assisted reproductive techniques in women over 45, using her own eggs, are unsuccessful. For this reason, older women are often advised to consider using donor eggs. However the receptiveness of the uterus also plays a part in a successful pregnancy outcome, therefore even with healthy donor eggs, success rates are still lower in women over 45.

So what's the good news? The good news is that although you can't turn back the clock, there are ways in which you can help improve and maintain the health of your eggs at any age, increasing your personal chances of conception. So read on!

Men

Male fertility doesn't decline as markedly with age compared to women. Men can sometimes remain fertile their whole life, but, as with females, chances of conception does reduce with age. Although they may not like to admit it, about one third of all fertility problems are linked to men. Sperm quality naturally reduces as men age. Sperm quality not only impacts the ability to conceive but also the viability of the pregnancy; poor sperm quality increases the risk of miscarriage.

However, again there is good news. Good nutrition, or lack there of, directly impacts sperm quality and potency and can assist in countering or accelerating the ageing process. Older men with a high intake of antioxidant nutrients including vitamin C, vitamin E and zinc, showed significantly reduced levels of sperm damage compared to men of same age and those with the highest intake of these nutrients showed levels of sperm damage comparable to those of much younger men. Page 64 outlines exactly what steps you can take to optimise your sperm health at any age.

"Hope is a renewable option: If you run out of it at the end of the day, you get to start over in the morning."

~ *Anonymous*

WEIGHT

Women

Maintaining a healthy weight is vitally important for fertility. Being overweight or underweight reduces your chances of conception. This has been confirmed in numerous studies dating back to the 1920's.

> RESEARCH SHOW THAT EXCESS BODY FAT HAS A SIGNIFICANT IMPACT ON FERTILITY AND THE ABILITY TO MAINTAIN A PREGNANCY BY:
> ✓ Disturbing ovulation, leading to irregular or lack of ovulation (anovulation)
> ✓ Contributing to heavy and/ or prolonged menstruation
> ✓ Reducing response to fertility medications
> ✓ Increasing the risk of gestational diabetes and pre-eclampsia

A BMI greater than 25 increases infertility, miscarriage risk and antenatal complications

A BMI greater than 31 increases the risk of having a child with neural tube defects, central nervous system complications, cardiovascular complications and digestive disturbances.

In a clinical trial, women attending an IVF clinic were put on a diet and exercise program for 6 months, whilst ceasing IVF treatment. Results showed an average weight loss of 10.2kg. Following the weight loss 90% of women who were previously not ovulating, spontaneously began to ovulate, 18 conceived naturally and 34 conceived after IVF treatment. Miscarriage rate dropped from 75% in the same group previously to 18% after the progam.

However the reverse is also true. Underweight women (classed as a BMI under 18.5) are more than twice as likely to take more than a year to fall pregnant. This is largely due to low body weight affecting healthy ovulation.

Men

Being overweight or underweight can also impact male fertility. Excess weight can lead to an increase in circulating estrogen in the body, which has a direct impact on spermatogenesis.

Studies confirm that male obesity is associated with lower sperm concentration, lower sperm count, lower levels of motile sperm, poor sperm morphology and increases in DNA damage. In a study of couples undergoing IVF treatment, men with normal BMI were found to have higher sperm concentration than overweight or obese men. A larger number of morbidly obese men also required prescribed fertility drugs to help achieve fertilization.

The good news is that recent studies show positive improvements in total sperm count and sperm volume after a weight loss.

Although less common in men, being underweight can also negatively impact sperm count and motility.

SMOKING

Women

Women who smoke are at least 1.5 times more likely to have fertility issues and take longer than a year to fall pregnant. This is also the case for those who are passive smokers compared to those in smoke free environments. Cigarette smoking is associated with reduced fertility, poor reproductive outcomes and a higher risk of IVF failure. Studies show that all reproductive functions are affected by smoking including impaired ovarian reserve, fallopian tube function and embryo development as well as increased menstrual irregularities. Nicotine has shown to negatively impact the production of luteinising hormone (LH), which is vital for ovulation. If fertilisation does occur, smoking may also affect the placenta, reducing the flow of nutrients and removal of toxins to and from the developing foetus as well as increasing the risk of early miscarriage. Smoke compounds can be found in ovarian tissue, uterine fluid and in the embryo, indicating a direct toxic affect.

Men

Smoking negatively affects sperm motility and seminal fluid quality. These negative effects have been shown to increase, the more cigarettes smoked. A recent study showed that only 6% of smokers had normal, healthy sperm parameters compared to 37% of non-smokers. Light smokers were found to have reduced sperm motility. Heavy smokers also showed reduced sperm motility as well as low sperm count and abnormally shaped sperm, all factors which can impair fertility.

The bottom line is that smokers, both male and female, are more likely to be infertile than non-smokers. The good news is that most of these negative effects have been found to reverse or greatly reduce within 12 smoke free months.

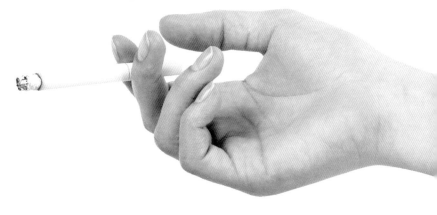

ALCOHOL

Women

I'm often asked, is it really that bad to have a few drinks when I'm trying to conceive? There are many conflicting opinions on this topic and the exact 'safe' limit, if there is such a thing, is extremely unclear. The facts we do know are that alcohol does have a negative effect on fertility and a growing baby, and that any amount of alcohol you consume will be passed onto your baby.

Alcohol interferes with the production of luteinising hormone (LH) and follicle stimulating hormone (FSH), both of which play a vital role in ovulation which is critical for there to be any possibility of conception. Alcohol intake during the week of conception can also increase the risk of early pregnancy loss.

For these reasons The National Health and Medical Research Council recommends that women who are trying to get pregnant should not drink at all because a 'no effect' level has not been established. Although the council does suggest that the risk associated with low-level drinking (such as one to two drinks per week) are likely to be low, they also acknowledge that this suggestion cannot be confirmed due to limitations of existing evidence.

So, the bottom line is that if you're serious about trying to get pregnant, it's best not to drink alcohol.

Men

Alcohol has been found to have a negative effect on all levels of the male reproductive system, with the most common symptom being abnormal or damaged sperm. Regular high alcohol consumption doubles the likelihood of low sperm count and presence of abnormal sperm. Alcohol consumption by both males and females during the week of conception has been found to increase the risk of early miscarriage.

In a study of the impact of high alcohol consumption on fertility, of the 100 alcoholics tested, only 12 showed normal sperm parameters. High alcohol consumption also reduces testosterone levels, which can lead to atrophy of the testes, impotence and infertility.

The National Health and Medical Research Council has not established any guidelines for men wishing to conceive. Standard guidelines for males recommends no more than 2 standard drinks on any one day and no more than 4 drinks on any single occasion. However the council also prefaced these guidelines by stating that no level of alcohol consumption can be guaranteed to be completely 'safe' or 'have no risk'.

CAFFEINE

Women

Cut down the coffee! A recent study showed that women who drink in excess of one cup of coffee per day are only half as likely to conceive as those who drink one cup or less per day. Women who drank more than 2-3 cups per day were nearly 5 times less likely to conceive compared to those who drink no coffee at all and chances of conception continue to decrease with increasing caffeine consumption. Caffeine intake can affect healthy ovulation and the function of the corpus luteum, both of which are critical for conception and the progression of a healthy pregnancy.

Increased caffeine consumption also increases this risk of early miscarriage. Women consuming more than 200mg of caffeine per day (about 2 cups of coffee) have double the risk of miscarriage compared to those consuming no caffeine.

Current recommendations suggest that women trying to conceive limit their caffeine intake to 100 – 200mg per day, which equates to 1 – 2 cups of regular coffee or 2 – 4 cups of regular black tea per day. It's also important to keep in mind that green tea, chocolate, hot chocolate and some soft drinks as well the array of new 'energy' drinks also contain caffeine, which can add up over the day. However in a study of patients undergoing IVF, women who consumed even modest amounts of caffeine (50mg per day) had decreased live birth rates.

So although the exact 'safe' intake is highly debatable, we do known that limiting or better still, eliminating caffeine from the diet positively affects fertility and healthy foetal development.

Men

Evidence of the impact of caffeine on male fertility is extremely limited and no 'safe' guidelines have been established. Most studies show that moderate intake has little to no impact on male fertility and that modest intake may even be helpful. However, studies do show that excessive intake negatively impacts sperm motility and the ability to achieve a healthy pregnancy. So although there are no specific 'safe' levels or 'upper safe limits' for males, experts agree that moderation is key.

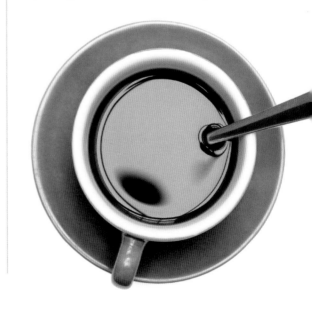

DIET/NUTRITION

Women

Experts agree that your prenatal nutrition has a direct effect on your ability to conceive and carry a healthy pregnancy and numerous studies dating back from the 1940s to today confirm this opinion. Even dating back to ancient times, women wishing to conceive were fed increased amount of nutrient rich foods. To some extent this is related to the impact of diet on weight and body fat however studies show that diet is a significant independent risk factor for infertility, regardless of body fat and BMI. This is due to the importance of diet in providing essential nutrients as well as being largely based on whole foods, avoiding chemical preservatives and additives.

The sooner healthy dietary changes are made, the better. As discussed on page 58 your eggs have a 90 day life cycle during which time you can influence the health of these developing eggs. So ideally healthy diet and lifestyle changes should be incorporated at least 3 months to a year before conceiving. In further chapters, I will discuss in more detail nutritional and dietary guidelines for specific reproductive health conditions and the 90 day fertility diet outlined on page 84 will help get you on the right track to conceiving your precious baby.

Men

While the impact of diet on female fertility is widely known, the impact of good nutrition on male fertility should not be underestimated. Studies confirm a direct link between sperm health and diet. As with women, this is linked to both excess body fat as well as lack of essential nutrients and increased exposure to artificial additives and preservatives. Sperm also follow a 90 day lifecycle. During this growth period you can positively and negatively impact sperm health through diet.

On page 70 I provide further detail about the best dietary modifications to improve sperm health of overall fertility. The 90 day fertility diet can also be of great benefit for men to increase chances of conception and the progression of a healthy pregnancy.

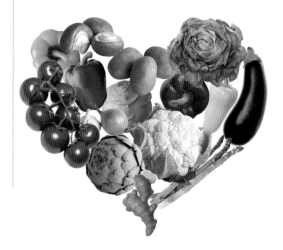

EXERCISE

Women

Too much, or too little exercise, will both negatively impact fertility. Women participating in regular high intensity, strenuous exercise show increased cortisol levels (as found in those with high stress levels) and reduced thyroid hormones. On top of this, excessive exercise also impacts estrogen and progesterone balance. High impact training can reduce the body's ability to produce progesterone, which is critical for ovulation. Extremely athletic women also have greatly reduced levels of body fat. Low body fat has a direct impact on estrogen production, reducing estrogen levels, which can lead to irregular or complete loss of the menstrual cycle as well as irregular or absence of ovulation.

However, before you throw out your trainers, at the other extreme, very little exercise will also negatively impact your ability to conceive. Just as women with very little body fat, may suffer from reduced estrogen production, those with excess body fat may experience increased estrogen production. This can have the same effect on the menstrual cycle, causing irregular of loss of periods as well as irregular or lack of ovulation. Also, just as regular strenuous activity can increase cortisol levels, lack of exercise can also increase cortisol levels. Regular exercise aids the body's natural stress response, improving our ability to deal with stress as well as helping to reduce cortisol levels.

Page 55 goes into more detail about the best exercise to help boost fertility for women.

Men

Sedentary lifestyle and lack of exercise reduces fertility in men, largely due to the influence on body fat levels, which can lead to impaired sperm production.

However, unlike women, men don't appear to be as affected by high intensity exercise. High-level exercise does appear to alter male hormonal balance. Short, intense bursts of exercise, appears to temporarily increase testosterone levels, whereas prolonged exercise (and to some extent in the hours following short bursts of exercise) appears to suppress testosterone levels. The extra heat produced during exercise is also not beneficial for sperm health. So although endurance training does appear to have a similar suppressive effect on the reproductive system in males, and some endurance athletes do present with non-specific modifications in sperm count, morphology and motility, it's not clear whether this has a clinically relevant effect on male reproduction.

Page 70 goes into more detail about the best exercise to help boost fertility for men.

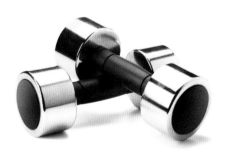

Medications

NOTE - If you or your partner are currently taking any of the following medications, please consult your Health Care Professional about potential impact on fertility, or reducing, changing or ceasing these medications.

WOMEN

Selective serotonin reuptake inhibitors (SSRI's)

Eg. Prozac, Zoloft, Paxil

SSRI's are prescribed for the treatment of depression and anxiety and there is much debate about their use during both the preconception period and during pregnancy. SSRI's don't directly impact the menstrual cycle or ovulation and have been listed as safe during this period.

However, SSRI's have been linked to higher rates of miscarriage, preterm birth, pregnancy complications as well as birth defects and long-term behavioural issues in the child as well as affecting the efficacy of infertility treatment.

Women with a history of depression are twice as likely to struggle with infertility and for this reason SSRI's are sometimes prescribed, under the understanding that the benefit outweighs the risk. However there is little evidence that women struggling with infertility benefit from the use of SSRI's and there is no evidence of improved pregnancy outcomes.

Tricyclic antidepressants (TCA's)

Eg. Amitriptyline, Amoxapine, Doxepin, Elavil

Tricyclic antidepressants are an older form of antidepressants and are less commonly prescribed due to their high side effect profile. However they may be used when SSRI's are ineffective or in more extreme cases of depression. Unlike SSRI's, tricyclic antidepressants do impact hormone production by increasing levels of prolactin, which stimulates milk production. This impacts the normal ovulation. Therefore these medications are not recommended during the preconception or pregnancy period.

Corticosteroids

Eg. Cortisone, Prednisone, Prednisolone

These medications have strong anti-inflammatory properties and are prescribed for conditions such as asthma, eczema and injury. General prescribed use of these medications does not appear to negatively impact fertility, in fact low doses may be prescribed during fertility treatment. However regular, high dose use may interfere with your body's ability to produce luteinising hormone (LH) and follicle stimulating hormone (FSH), which can prevent ovulation from occurring.

Non-steroidal anti-inflammatories (NSAID's)

Eg. Nurofen, Advil (Ibuprofen), Naprogesic (Naproxen), Aspirin
Occasional use of these medications for mild pain does not appear to negatively impact fertility or conception however regular use of NSAID's can directly affect ovulation. Use of these medications has been linked to reduced ability for ovaries to release an egg at ovulation, leading to irregular or anovulation. Side effects have shown to reverse once treatment has stopped.

MEN

Selective serotonin reuptake inhibitors (SSRI's)

Eg. Prozac, Zoloft, Paxil
Prescribed in the treatment of depression and anxiety, SSRI's can have a significant impact on sperm production. Unlike women, where potential risks are still in debate, conclusive studies show that SSRI's have a detrimental effect on sperm production, sperm motility as well as sperm quality. Men taking SSRI's have been shown to have significantly reduced sperm concentration and percentage of normal sperm as well as a significantly increased percentage of sperm with DNA damage. This reduces both the ability to conceive as well as risk of miscarriage and birth defects. Other side effects include decreased libido, reduced ability to orgasm and ejaculate and erectile dysfunction.

Calcium channel blockers

Eg. Norvasc, Cardizem
Calcium channel blockers are prescribed for the treatment of high blood pressure, angina and irregular heartbeat, however they are generally not the first line treatment for these conditions. This type of medication can reduce the ability of sperm to fertilise the egg.

Tricyclic antidepressants (TCA's)

Eg. Endep, Placil, Dothep, Sinequan, Tofranil
Tricyclic antidepressants are less commonly prescribed in preference to the newer SSRI's, however both forms of anti-depressant medications directly impact sperm health.

Ketoconazole

Eg. Nizoral, Extina, Xolegel
Ketoconazole is prescribed in the treatment of fungal infection. Whilst topical application within creams, ointments or powders does not appear to impact fertility, oral ingestion of ketoconazole tablets can decrease testosterone and sperm production. Use of this medication is generally for the acute treatment of infection and side effects appear to reverse once use is discontinued.

Non-steroidal anti-inflammatories (NSAID's)

Eg. Nurofen, Advil (Ibuprofen), Naprogesic (Naproxen), Aspirin
Unlike women, men do not appear to suffer any negative reproductive effects from the use of NSAID's.

Other medications such as antipsychotics, cancer medications, prostate medications as well as some antibiotics can also negatively impact fertility in both men and women.

Health conditions

MENSTRUAL CYCLE IRREGULARITIES – WHEN THINGS AREN'T 'NORMAL'

A regular menstrual period is a sign of good health. It indicates that your body is healthy enough to nourish a growing baby. Although there can be significant difference is what is 'normal' for every women, there are some irregularities that can interfere with fertility.

Ammenorhoea

It's quite normal for women to experience 1 or 2 missed periods. This is often due to stress or acute illness and generally rectifies itself. However if you miss more than 3 consecutive periods, this should be investigated.

LACK OF MENSTRUATION CAN BE CAUSED BY:

Nutritional deficiencies
Lack of iron and zinc in particular as well as vitamin C and B vitamins can affect menstruation. Tests can be done to assess your levels and supplementation has been shown to help correct deficiencies.

Stress
Acute stress can cause the temporary loss of your period. However when the stress is prolonged and chronic, this can lead to a longer-term loss of menstruation and impaired fertility. Steps should be undertaken to reduce stress levels and help support the return of a regular cycle. Page 56 goes into more detail about strategies to reduce chronic stress.

Overweight/Underweight
Being substantially overweight or underweight can lead to amenorrhoea. This relates to high or low BMI as well as body fat levels. Even those with a 'normal' BMI who have an extremely high muscle mass and low body fat may also experience lack of menstruation. These factors can be positively influenced by healthy diet and exercise.

PCOS
Amenorrhoea can be a symptom of Polycystic ovarian syndrome.

Thyroid imbalance

Loss of the menstrual cycle can be a symptom of an overactive thyroid (hyperthyroidism). This is discussed in further detail on page 39

Short cycles

Short menstrual cycles can indicate a lack of ovulation or a shortened luteal phase. A short luteal phase, (known as luteal phase defect) is assessed as less than 10 - 12 days. This doesn't allow sufficient time for full development of the endometrium. This can mean the fertilised egg doesn't properly implant or may miscarry shortly after implantation.

The most common cause of a luteal phase defect is lack of progesterone. Although there is no specific diagnostic test for luteal phase defects, the length of your luteal phase can be assessed using the charting tools outlined on page 8 and tracking the days from ovulation to the commencement of your next menstrual cycle. Your doctor may also perform blood tests to assess follicle-stimulating hormone (FSH) levels, luteinising hormone (LH) levels and progesterone levels or in some cases an endometrial biopsy may be performed.

Luteal phase defects can be treated using prescribed medications such as progesterone tablets or injections, human chorionic gonadotropin, or clomid. Alternatively vitex-agnus castus (outlined in further detail on page 51 is a herb with progesterone stimulating properties, which has been found to be an effective natural treatment especially when combined with vitamin B6.

Long or/heavy periods

Long or heavy periods can be a sign of hormonal imbalance and/or a failure to ovulate. This is generally related to a high estrogen to progesterone balance. Healthy progesterone levels are necessary for ovulation and conception as well as helping to stop excess bleeding during your period. Bleeding which continues longer than normal or is heavier than normal can indicate low progesterone or a low progesterone to estrogen balance (estrogen dominance). Your Doctor may prescribe medication to help rectify any imbalance. You can also assist natural hormonal balance by supporting the excretion of excess estrogen via the liver through diet and herbal support and using herbal treatment to help correct underlying imbalance.

Thick, dark, brownish menstrual bleeding or clots

Healthy menstrual flow should be free flowing and bright red in colour. Menstrual flow that is dark or brown in colour or contains clots can be old blood left over from the previous cycle. This can be caused by poor uterine circulation, sluggish menstrual flow or poor uterine tone. Following a healthy diet, such as outlined in the 90 day fertility diet, and keeping well hydrated and active will help to improve circulation and blood flow.

POLYCYSTIC OVARIAN SYNDROME (PCOS)

Spotting

Spotting can be a regular occurrence for some women and often times it's no cause for concern.

HOWEVER IN SOME CASES IT CAN BE A SIGN OF AN UNDERLYING CONDITION SUCH AS:
- ✓ Failure to ovulate (or some women also experience spotting at the time of ovulation)
- ✓ Hormonal imbalance
- ✓ Excessive exercise
- ✓ Poor diet/nutrition
- ✓ Cervical abnormalities
- ✓ Ovarian cysts
- ✓ Endometriosis

Therefore if you do experience spotting and are trying to conceive, you should advise your Health Care Professional.

PCOS is a relatively common yet extremely complex condition. The exact cause is largely unknown but is believed to have a genetic component, being commonly found in mothers, daughters and sisters.

THE COMMON PRESENTATION OF PCOS INCLUDES:
- ✓ Polycystic ovaries (multiple ovarian cysts)
- ✓ Menstrual irregularities or amenorrhoea
- ✓ Anovulation or irregular ovulation
- ✓ Heavy menstrual bleeding
- ✓ PMS/PMT
- ✓ High androgen levels (male hormone) low ovarian estrogen
- ✓ Excess hair around the face, nipples, navel and pubic area
- ✓ Acne
- ✓ Weight gain/Obesity
- ✓ Insulin resistance/poor blood sugar regulation
- ✓ Reduced fertility or infertility

However not all women diagnosed with PCOS will present with all of the above symptoms. You may even have polycystic ovaries yet not have any symptoms of PCOS. PCOS can have a severe or mild presentation with some women unaware they have the condition. If you have concerns as to whether you have PCOS, it's important to consult with your Health Care Professional to get a proper diagnosis.

There is no specific diagnostic test for PCOS. If your Health Care Professional suspects that you might have PCOS they may take the following steps to help reach a diagnosis:

Menstrual History
You will be asked about your menstrual cycle, any irregularities, heavy bleeding or changes in weight.

Physical examination
YOUR HEALTH CARE PROFESSIONAL WILL:
- ✓ Take your blood pressure
- ✓ Check your weight and BMI
- ✓ Measure your waist circumference
- ✓ Check for increased hair growth (of you use any form of hair removal for excess hair, this should be mentioned).
- ✓ Palpate your pelvic region to asses any potential swelling in the area caused by cysts on your ovaries

---

Blood tests
A blood test may be recommended to asses for increased androgen levels and check your blood sugar levels.

Ultrasound/Sonogram
Ultrasound may be performed to visually asses the presentation or number of cysts on your ovaries and examine your endometrium, which may be thicker than normal.

Treatment

Balancing hormones

Medications
Progesterone
Either on its own or within the Pill, is often prescribed to help regulate the menstrual cycle, balance hormones and minimise symptoms.

Clomiphene Citrate (Clomid)
Is commonly prescribed to stimulate ovulation in women with PCOS who are trying to conceive and may not be ovulating.

Herbs
Peony
Peony is beneficial in the treatment of PCOS for its ability to help reduce androgen (male hormone) levels and regulate estrogen and progesterone production. This herb works well when combined with liquorice.

Vitex
Vitex helps stimulate ovulation which can help improve chances of conception in those with erratic or anovulation.

Herbs should not be self-prescribed. See your natural fertility specialist or other qualified health care professional for specific dose recommendations.

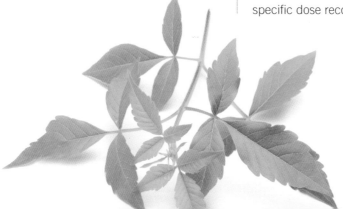

Supporting healthy blood sugar regulation

The insulin resistance component of PCOS is a significant contributing factor in infertility. Poor insulin control directly affects your fertility and ability to conceive. It can disturb normal ovulation and increase the risk of miscarriage. For this reason, Gynaecologists may prescribe medications to helps stabilise blood sugar but much can be done to support insulin resistance and healthy blood sugar levels through diet alone.

Medications

Metformin

Is commonly prescribed for people with type 2 diabetes as well as women with PCOS. Metformin helps control the amount of glucose in the bloodstream. Speak with your doctor about the benefits, risks and side effects of this medication.

Diet

Low GI

Eating a low glycaemic index (GI) diet helps to reduce insulin demand and support healthy stable blood sugar levels. Low GI foods break down slowly in the body releasing sustained energy and don't cause the dramatic spike and subsequent drop in blood sugar caused by high GI foods such as refined carbohydrates and sugars. A study in the Medical Journal of Metabolism concluded that a low carbohydrate, high protein diet helped insulin resistance and a high carbohydrate, low protein diet made insulin resistance worse. Although it's not necessary to completely cut out carbohydrates, reducing the consumption of refined carbohydrates and replacing these with wholegrain alternatives such as wholemeal breads, quinoa, millet and brown rice as well as increasing your protein will help reduce the insulin load.

High fibre

High fibre diets further support blood sugar balance by slowing the absorption of sugar into the blood stream, reducing the insulin spike. Fibre also supports healthy estrogen metabolism and reduction of androgens.

Small regular meals

A healthy PCOS diet should include 3 balanced meals and 2 healthy snacks eaten at regular intervals throughout the day. This helps to maintain healthy blood sugar levels and reduces sugar cravings.

Oily fish, nuts, seeds and other sources of essential fatty acids

Essential fatty acids also help to lower the GI of foods and help further support healthy blood sugar levels.

Nutrients

Chromium

Chromium is a trace mineral that supports insulin activity. Clinical studies have shown improved insulin sensitivity in women with PCOS using chromium. Chromium can also be safely taken throughout pregnancy and breastfeeding.

Recommended dose – 1000mcg per day

Food sources – Broccoli, barley, oats, green beans, tomatoes, romaine lettuce

Vitamin D

Vitamin D deficiency is commonly found in women presenting with insulin resistance or diabetes. Studies show that deficiency may play a role in blood sugar balance as well as increase the risk of developing insulin resistance, diabetes and gestational diabetes. Further studies are currently being conducted to confirm the exact mechanism of action of vitamin D in blood sugar regulation.

Recommended dose – 1000mcg per day
Recommended dose – 1000IU per day

Food sources – Milk, butter, salmon, tuna, cod liver oil, halibut liver oil, prawns, eggs yolk.

The richest natural source of vitamin D is from sunlight.

Herbs

Gymnema

- Gymnema has been used for centuries in the management of blood glucose. It supports healthy blood glucose levels by regulating the absorption of sugar. It achieves this by acting on the pancreatic cells, which produce insulin, to help enable more efficient insulin production as well as stimulating the production of the enzymes that help uptake glucose from the blood stream into cells. Several studies have proved Gymnema to be as effective as medications in the treatment of diabetes and insulin resistance and it is commonly prescribed by medical practitioners in Europe. This traditional herb also helps reduce sugar cravings and supports healthy weight loss.
- Gymnema should only be used to help reduce symptoms prior to pregnancy and should not be used during pregnancy or breastfeeding.

Recommended dose – 200 – 400mg 3 times per day

Cinnamon

- You probably recognise this herb from your favorite cake or muffin recipe. Now clinical studies show that therapeutic doses of this aromatic spice have a strong balancing effect on blood sugar levels, greatly improving diabetic symptoms. Long before the blood sugar regulating properties of cinnamon were discovered cinnamon was used traditionally for centuries to help reduce heavy menstrual bleeding and as a warming tonic for a 'cold' uterus. The term 'cold' uterus is a term used to describe a congested uterus with poor circulation and menstrual irregularities. It also acts as a warming, digestive tonic. You can freely use this spice for cooking during all phases of conception, pregnancy and breastfeeding.
- However therapeutic doses of cinnamon should only be used to help reduce symptoms prior to pregnancy and should not be used during pregnancy or breastfeeding.

Recommended dose – 1000mg 3 times per day

Exercise

Exercise is beneficial for general health and fertility and is particularly beneficial to help promote weight loss and maintenance of a healthy weight in women with PCOS. Exercise helps improve insulin sensitivity and boost metabolism. A combination of aerobic and resistance exercise has been found to work best.

The low GI and high fibre basis of the 90 day fertility diet at the end of this book is ideal for those with PCOS.

ENDOMETRIOSIS

The endometrium normally resides in the uterus, forming the uterine lining, and is expelled and rebuilt each month during menstruation. Endometriosis is a condition in which endometrial tissue grows outside the uterus, most commonly on the ovaries, in the fallopian tubes, the outer wall of the uterus, the ligaments of the uterus or ovaries, in the bowel, the ureters or the bladder. Endometriosis does also occur less commonly in other areas of the body.

The displaced endometrial tissue responds and performs in the same way as the uterine lining. The tissue builds up as the body moves towards ovulation and then breaks down and bleeds during menstruation. This bleeding can trigger inflammation and pain and over time can lead to scarring, known as adhesions. Endometriosis has a significant impact on fertility and is a causative factor in 35 – 50% of fertility issues in women.

The cause of endometriosis is largely unknown and symptoms can vary greatly.

MOST COMMON SYMPTOMS INCLUDE:
- ✓ Severe period pain (or pain may last all month long)
- ✓ Lower abdominal pain or back pain
- ✓ Heavy bleeding and/or clotting
- ✓ Abnormally long or short cycles
- ✓ PMS
- ✓ PMT
- ✓ Painful intercourse
- ✓ Abdominal swelling
- ✓ Infertility

As these symptoms are somewhat vague and can occur without the presence of endometriosis, some women are not aware they have the condition until it's discovered during unrelated surgery. Therefore diagnosis and prevention can be difficult. However endometriosis does appear to have a genetic connection and is commonly seen in mothers, daughters and sisters. Endometriosis is also found to be associated with a relative estrogen to progesterone excess. Speak to your Health Care Professional if you are concerned about whether you may have Endometriosis.

Treatment

Surgery

Most diagnoses occurring during a laparoscopy, when gynaecologists can see the misplaced endometrial tissue. During this procedure, small incisions are made between the navel and the pubic bone, through which a thin instrument with fibre optics is inserted so the surgeon can view the inner organs. The exact location of the incisions depends on your surgeons experience and your unique presentation. Sometimes a laparoscopy is simply performed as a diagnostic tool, or in more severe cases, endometrial tissue as well as any scar tissue and adhesions can be removed or reduced in attempts to improve fertility or reduce related symptoms. Unfortunately removal is not necessarily the magic bullet cure we'd like it to be, as endometrial tissue can grow back over time. However following the natural approaches outlined below can help reduce regrowth.

Balancing hormones

Medications
The Pill, Gonadotrophin-releasing hormone agonist, Progestin, Danazol

These medications help to correct hormonal imbalance. The aim of these treatments, are to reduce the excess estrogen in relation to progesterone. This helps to slow or prevent further growth of displaced tissue and reduce symptoms. These medications are also contraceptives, blocking conception, and are therefore not able to be used when trying to conceive.

Herbs
Vitex

Vitex is one of the most commonly used herbs, prescribed for its progesterone enhancing action. This helps to rebalance the estrogen dominance associated with endometriosis (refer to page 51 for full overview).

Natural progesterone cream

Natural progesterone creams are generally derived from either Wild Yam or soybeans. The active ingredient, diosgenin, in then synthesised into a molecular structure identical to human progesterone. These are sometimes referred to as 'human-identical' or 'bio-identical' progesterone. The cream is rubbed into the skin for absorption into the blood stream.

These herbs should not be self-prescribed. See your natural fertility specialist or other qualified health care professional for dose recommendations.

Reducing congestion and inflammation

The excess endometrial tissue leads to a great deal of congestion within the reproductive system. Every month as bleeding occurs scar tissue builds up, further exacerbating this congestion.

Herbs
Calendula

Calendula is an excellent herb for improving lymphatic drainage and reducing internal congestion. It also helps to reduce muscle spasms and heavy menstrual bleeding as well as providing anti-inflammatory action. Calendula should only be used prior to conception under advisement of your health care professional.

Recommended dose – 1000 - 4000g dried flower as a tea 3 times per day or 0.5 - 1ml fluid extract 3 times per day.

Turmeric

Turmeric supports detoxification pathways to help further reduce congestion as well as imparting strong anti-inflammatory and antioxidant activity. Turmeric should only be used prior to conception under advise-ment of your health care professional.

Recommended dose – 400 - 600mg 3 times per day

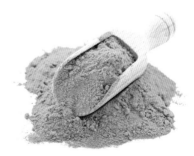

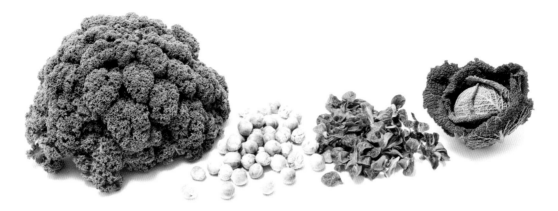

Nutrition

FOODS TO INCREASE

To help ease the congestion and inflammation associated with endometriosis your diet should focus on:

Fresh, organic fruits and vegetables
Fruits and vegetables should form the bulk of your diet. They are high in essential nutrients and aid in the reduction of inflammation. Cruciferous vegetables such as broccoli, kale, cauliflower, bok choy, brussel sprouts, cabbage, collards greens and mustard greens are particularly beneficial as the contain a nutrient known as diindolymethane which supports hormone balance by assisting in the breakdown of estrogen.

High fibre
Fibre helps cleanse the body, reducing congestion and also aiding in the excretion of excess estrogen.

Oily fish, nuts, seeds and other sources of essential fatty acids
Essential fatty acids help reduce the inflammation and pain associated with endometriosis.

The 90 day fertility diet outlined in this book combines these principles and has been specifically designed to help reduce inflammation and congestion and support fertility, conception and the progression of a healthy pregnancy.

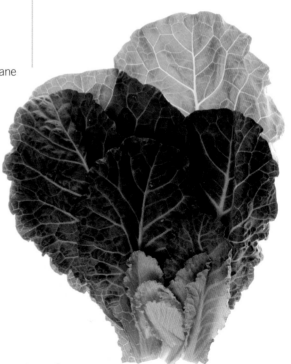

FOODS TO DECREASE

In cases of endometriosis it's also important to avoid foods that have been shown to exacerbate inflammation and congestion, these include:

Wheat and gluten

Studies have linked high wheat intake with increased pain in endometriosis. Gluten sensitivity and intolerance have also been found to be more common in women with endometriosis. For this reason I recommend removing wheat (ideally all forms of gluten) from the diet for 2 months to see if it reduces symptoms.

Red meat

Red meat can exacerbate inflammation and although doesn't need to be removed from the diet, it should be limited to 3 times per week or less. Ideally meat should be organic. Studies also suggest minimising ham and pork intake.

Dairy

Dairy can contribute to congestion within the body, with popular homogenised, pasteurised cow's milk being one of the hardest dairy products to digest and most congestive. The best forms of dairy to consume are organic natural yogurts and where possible choose milk alternatives such as almond, rice or oat milk.

Toxins

Toxins of all forms increase the detoxification load on the body, contributing to increased congestion and inflammation.

TO MINIMISE YOUR TOXIC
LOAD YOU SHOULD:
✓ Eat organic
✓ Use organic body products and make-up
✓ Use eco-friendly, low chemical detergents and cleaning products
✓ Use natural feminine hygiene products
✓ Avoid all exposure to pesticides, herbicides and synthetic fertilisers

Following the 90 day fertility diet at the end of this book is an ideal way to help reduce symptoms and support conception for those with endometriosis.

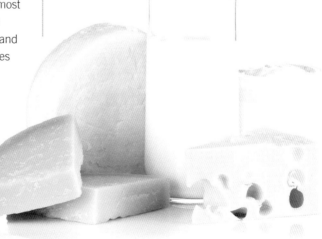

THYROID

Thyroid issues are complicated conditions that can have a significant impact on fertility. Below is an outline of medical and alternative treatments, however any thyroid concerns should be discussed with your Health Care Professional and should not be self-treated.

HYPOTHYROIDISM

Hypothyroidism (low thyroid function or underactive thyroid) is one of the leading causes of infertility or early miscarriage. Underactive thyroid is associated with reduced FSH and LH levels, which are vital for egg maturation and ovulation as well as regulation of estrogen and progesterone. It's a relatively common condition, which can often go undiagnosed. Although most studies focus largely on thyroid imbalance and female fertility, a recent literature review confirmed that thyroid function can also impacts male fertility.

SYMPTOMS CAN VARY BUT INCLUDE:
✓ Tiredness/fatigue
✓ Depression, irritability
✓ Constipation or slow transit time
✓ Weight gain and/or difficulty losing weight
✓ Dry skin hair and nails
✓ Hair loss
✓ Eczema
✓ Slow pulse rate
✓ Shortness of breath

✓ Low body temperature and intolerance to cold
✓ Muscle cramps
✓ Low libido
✓ Irregular menstrual cycles
✓ Swollen thyroid (goiter)
✓ Difficulty conceiving or recurrent miscarriage

If you are having difficulty conceiving suffer 3 or more of the above symptoms, I advise speaking with your Health Care Professional about thyroid tests.

Treatment

Medications

Levothyroxine (L-Thyroxine)
Eg. Levoxyl, Synthroid, Levothroid
Levothyroxine provides thyroid hormone when the thyroid is under functioning or inactive.

Surgery

Surgery is rarely required for hypothyroidism and is only performed where there is presence of large goiters that are impacting esophageal function or potential cancerous lesions.

Herbal support

The adrenals are under extra strain when the thyroid is over or under functioning.

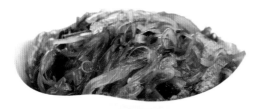

Herbal treatments are an excellent supportive adjunct for both adrenal function and stress levels.

Kelp

Is a good natural source of iodine and other essential minerals. However it's important not to take too much iodine, therefore kelp should not be taken with iodine supplements unless under the supervision of your Health Care Professional. Only high quality kelp supplements should be used as some have been found to contain high levels of toxins as found in certain seawater.

> Recommended dose – providing 220mcg iodine per day

Withania

(Indian ginseng)

Withania helps reduce high cortisol levels associated with stress and adrenal dysfunction.

> Recommended dose – 3000mg – 9000mg per day

Oats

Oats are a nourishing tonic for the nervous system, aiding in the reduction or cortisol levels.

> Recommended dose – 1000 – 4000mg 3 times per day

Liquorice

Liquorice is generally used in combination with other adrenal herbs. It provides mild anti-inflammatory action, acts as an immune system regulator as well as nourishing the nervous system. You may find much information about liquorice raising blood pressure, however this is only in high doses.

> Recommended dose – 300mg – 1000mg per day in a blend as prescribed by your Health Care Practitioner

Nutritional support

Iodine

Iodine is required for the production of thyroid hormone and is also required for brain development during pregnancy. However, speak to your Health Care Professional before taking iodine if you are already taking thyroid medication.

> Recommended dose – 220 – 250mcg per day
>
> Food sources – Seaweed and sea vegetables, fish, shellfish, yoghurt, cow's milk, eggs, mozzarella cheese

Selenium

Selenium supports the function of several enzymes involved in thyroid function. Selenium also provides potent antioxidant activity.

> Recommended dose – 60mcg per day
>
> Food sources – Brazil nuts (highest known source), crab, tuna, lobster, meat, wheat, soybean

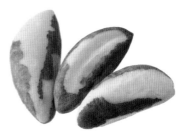

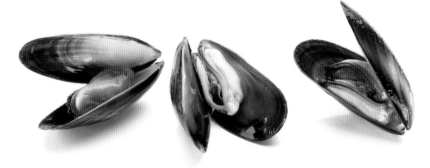

Zinc

Zinc is involved in many metabolic processes within the thyroid and is also essential for healthy immune function and ovulation.

Recommended dose – 11mg per day

Food sources – Oysters, shellfish, red meat, pork, chicken, eggs, hard cheese, nuts, pulses, wholegrains

Vitamin B12

Vitamin B12 deficiency is common in women with hypothyroidism and is also important for many metabolic functions.

Recommended dose – 500mg per day

Food sources – Trout, beef, clams, kidney, crab, oysters, lamb, tuna, salmon, sardines, veal, milk, yoghurt, cheese, eggs

Antioxidants

Vitamins A, C and E provide excellent antioxidant support for healthy thyroid function. The safest supplemental form of vitamin A is beta-carotene, which can safely be taken throughout pregnancy.

Recommended dose – Beta-carotene –3000 – 6000mcg per day

Vitamin C – 50 – 500mg per day per day

Vitamin E – 50 – 200IU (33 – 133mg) per day

Antioxidant rich food sources – Blueberries, black-berries, raspberries, goji berries, broccoli, tomatoes, green leafy vegetables, brightly coloured foods

Fish Oil - Omega 3

Omega 3 helps reduce inflammation and can be beneficial during pre-conception and pregnancy. Fish Oil is the best source of Omega 3 for hypothyroid as flaxseeds may have mild thyroid suppressive properties, therefore should be avoided. The DHA component of fish oil is the most important.

Recommended dose – 300mg – 500mg DHA

Food sources – Salmon, sardines, halibut, snapper, tuna, scallops, shrimp, cod, red fish, white fish

Diet and lifestyle

✓ Diet should focus on whole foods with a large vegetable base
✓ Reduce refined processed foods such as white bread and pasta
✓ Limit red meat and deli meats
✓ Increase fish and vegetarian proteins such as tofu and legumes
✓ Eliminate trans fatty acids found in processed foods
✓ Limit alcohol and caffeine intake
✓ Aim to exercise for 30 minutes 5 days a week

The 90 day fertility diet at the end of this book is ideal for those with thyroid conditions.

HYPERTHYROIDISM

Hyperthyroidism (overactive thyroid) can also reduce fertility. An overactive thyroid leads to an overproduction of thyroid hormones.

SYMPTOMS OF HYPERTHYROIDISM ARE WIDE AND VARIED BUT INCLUDE:
- ✓ Weight loss with no change in diet or exercise routine
- ✓ Increased appetite
- ✓ Anxiety, irritability
- ✓ Sleep disturbance/difficulty sleeping
- ✓ Tremors in your hands and fingers
- ✓ Rapid or irregular heartbeat or palpitations (noticeable pounding of your heart)
- ✓ Increased sweating
- ✓ Increased sensitivity to heat
- ✓ Menstrual irregularities/ amenorrhoea
- ✓ Frequent bowel movements
- ✓ Loss of libido
- ✓ Fatigue/muscle weakness

If you are having difficulty conceiving and suffer 3 or more of the above symptoms, I advise speaking with your Health Care Professional about thyroid tests.

Treatment

Medications

Liquid radioactive iodine
A single dose of liquid radioactive iodine is sometimes prescribed to suppress an overactive thyroid. However, up to half of patients who receive this treatment experience permanent hypothyroid within a year of treatment.

Anti-thyroid medications
These medications have a suppressive effect on the thyroid gland, reducing overproduction of thyroid hormone. Treatment will generally start to improve symptoms within 2 – 3 months and is medication is continued for at least a year. This may be a permanent cure for some people or others may relapse. These medications can affect the liver and liver damage is a common side effect of these medications.

Beta-blockers
Usually prescribed in the treatment of high blood pressure, these medications may be used to help reduce rapid heart rate and palpitations. They do not however reduce overactive thyroid.

Surgery

Thyroidectomy may be performed in some cases. This involves removing part or most of the thyroid gland. This is only an option in a few cases. There are risks involved including potential damage to neighbouring organs and lifelong medications will be required to supply the body with adequate thyroid hormone.

Herbal support

The adrenals are often overloaded when the thyroid is over or under functioning. Herbal treatments can be very supportive for both adrenal function and stress levels.

Lemon Balm
(Melissa officianalis)
Lemon balm is helps calm and reduce stress levels as well as helping to normalise overactive thyroid function. This herb is one of the most beneficial for thyroid function however it has not been proven safe during pregnancy and therefore should only be used under the supervision of your Health Care Professional when trying to conceive.

Recommended dose – 300 – 500mg
3 times per day

Oats
Oats are a nourishing tonic for the nervous system, aiding in the reduction or cortisol levels.

Recommended dose – 1000 – 4000mg
3 times per day

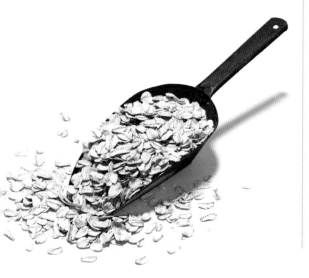

Withania somnifera/ Indian ginseng
Withania helps reduce high cortisol levels associated with stress and adrenal dysfunction.

Recommended dose – 3000mg – 9000mg per day

Liquorice
Liquorice is generally used in combination with other adrenal herbs. It provides mild anti-inflammatory action, immune system regulator as well as nourishing the nervous system. You may find much information about liquorice raising blood pressure, however this is only in high doses.

Recommended dose – 300mg – 1000mg per day in a blend as prescribed by your Health Care Practitioner

Nutritional support

Fish Oil/Flaxseed Oil - Omega 3
Omega 3 may be useful to help reduce inflammation associated with hyperthyroidism. Fish Oil is the strongest source of omega 3, however flaxseeds may possess mild thyroid suppressive properties, therefore both can be beneficial.

Recommended dose – 3000mg - 20,000mg per day (1tsp – 1 tbsp per day)

Food sources – salmon, tuna, flaxseeds, flaxseed meal, flaxseed oil

L-carnitine
L-carnitine has been shown to have a mild suppressive action on an overactive thyroid.

Recommended dose – 2000 – 4000mg per day

Food sources – Beef, chicken, codfish, milk, cheese

Antioxidants

Antioxidant nutrients including vitamin A, C, E, alpha-lipoic acid and selenium can help to protect and support the thyroid and other organs from oxidative damage. Beta-carotene is the best supplemental source of vitamin A when trying to conceive as it can be safely taken throughout pregnancy.

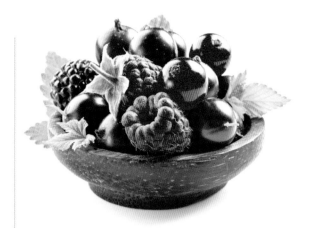

Recommended dose - Beta-carotene - 3000 – 6000mcg per day Vitamin C – 50 – 500mg per day per day

Vitamin E – 50 – 200IU (33 – 133mg) per day

Alpha-lipoic acid – Selenium – 60mcg per day

Antioxidant rich food sources – Blueberries, blackberries, raspberries, goji berries, broccoli, tomatoes, green leafy vegetables, brightly coloured foods

Vitamin D

Vitamin D is a common deficiency. It helps support immune function and reduce inflammation.

Recommended dose – 1000IU per day

Food sources – Milk, butter, salmon, tuna, cod liver oil, halibut liver oil, prawns, eggs yolk.

The richest natural source of vitamin D is from sunlight.

Probiotics

A probiotic containing lactobacillus acidophilus can help support digestive health and reduce inflammation caused by dietary allergens or poor digestion.

Recommended dose – 10 – 50 billion per day

Food sources – Yoghurt (naturally set), cottage cheese, buttermilk, miso, tempeh, kefir

Diet and lifestyle

✓ Dietary allergens can increase inflammation so eliminate any suspected allergenic foods. The most common allergenic foods are dairy, wheat (gluten), soy, corn, preservatives and additives. Your Health Care Professional may wish to run an allergy test.

✓ Aim for whole foods and reduce refined processed foods such as white bread and pasta

✓ Increase vegetable intake, particularly cruciferous vegetables

✓ Limit red meat and processed meats

✓ Increase fish and vegetarian proteins such as tofu and legumes

✓ Eliminate trans fatty acids found in processed foods

✓ Limit alcohol and caffeine intake

✓ Aim to exercise for 30 minutes 5 days a week

PELVIC INFLAMMATORY DISEASE (PID)

Pelvic Inflammatory Disease is an infection of the female reproductive organs most commonly resulting from sexually transmitted disease. 90% of cases are caused by untreated chlamydia or gonorrhoea. PID occurs when the disease causing organisms, originally transmitted into the cervix, are left untreated and allowed to travel from the cervix to the upper genital tract. Other causes of PID include abortion, use of IUD, childbirth and pelvic surgery.

Chlamydia is one of the most insidious infections to cause PID, often presenting with no symptoms. For this reason Chlamydia is commonly only discovered when a woman presents for investigations for her infertility. To help avoid this many GP's will request a chlamydia test as part of a general woman's health check-up or you can request the test from your GP yourself. However this initial blood test for chlamydia is not 100% accurate so if infection is suspected your GP may prescribe treatment anyway or run further diagnostic testing.

> THE SYMPTOMS OF PID MAY VARY, BUT INCLUDE:
> ✓ Abnormal vaginal discharge, yellow or green in colour and/or an unusual odour
> ✓ Heavier than usual periods
> ✓ Bleeding between periods
> ✓ Painful urination
> ✓ Dull pain or tenderness in the stomach, lower abdominal region or the upper right abdomen
> ✓ Fever or chills

> ✓ Nausea and vomiting
> ✓ Pain during intercourse or bleeding afterwards
> FERTILITY COMPLICATIONS INCLUDE:
> ✓ Scarring, damage or development of abscesses within the fallopian tubes
> ✓ Increased (about 1 in 10) risk of ectopic pregnancy
> ✓ Miscarriage
> ✓ Premature birth
> ✓ Stillbirth

For some women, the symptoms of PID will present rapidly and they will become quite unwell over the course of a few days. Sometimes the symptoms develop more slowly and are milder, often going unnoticed. For some women, there are no symptoms present at all. However, even with no symptoms you are still at risk of complications. The earlier treatment commences, the less chance of complications.

Treatment

Medications
Initial treatment of PID involves the prescription of antibiotics for at least 2 weeks, commonly up to 6 weeks, to clear up the infection.

Surgery
In more severe cases, PID can cause abscesses within the reproductive system. Theses require surgical removal to prevent them rupturing and spreading infection.

UTERINE FIBROIDS

Uterine fibroids are small, non-cancerous growths, which occur within the uterus also known as uterine leiomyomas or uterine myomata. They can vary in size from microscopic and quite unnoticeable to large growths that can put cause pressure and pain. Fibroids can grow within the muscles of the uterus, on the outside of the uterus, within the uterine cavity or on rare occasions may growth within the cervix.

THESE ARE CALLED:

Myometrial fibroids
Grow within the muscle wall of the uterus (myometrium)
Symptoms can include:
- ✧ Heavy menstrual bleeding if large in size
- ✧ Pressure on adjacent organs if especially large

Extra-uterine fibroids
These are attached to the outside surface of the uterus
Symptoms can include:
- ✧ Heavy menstrual bleeding if large in size
- ✧ May cause pressure related symptoms
- ✧ If found around the fallopian tubes, can interfere with fertility

Intra-uterine fibroids
Symptoms can include:
- ✧ Commonly cause heavy menstrual bleeding even if small
- ✧ Reduced fertility and increased risk of miscarriage due to the effect of the fibroid/s on the endometrium, affecting implantation

Fibroids generally appear after puberty within a woman's childbearing years when estrogen levels are high and commonly reduce after menopause. Although the cause is unknown, we do know that their growth is dependent on estrogen.

FACTORS THAT MAY INCREASE THE RISK OF FIBROID DEVELOPMENT INCLUDE:
- ✓ Increased exposure to estrogen due to estrogen dominance
- ✓ early menarche/puberty
- ✓ few or no pregnancies
- ✓ long follicular phase menstrual cycle
- ✓ hormone replacement therapy

FIBROIDS ARE BELIEVED TO CAUSE INFERTILITY IN AROUND 2 – 10% OF INFERTILITY CASES DUE TO THE FOLLOWING COMPLICATIONS:
- ✓ Irregular or lack of ovulation
- ✓ Blocked fallopian tubes
- ✓ Poor implantation due to endometrial disturbance
- ✓ Abnormal uterine blood flow hindering sperms journey to the egg

Not all women with fibroids will experience fertility issues in fact some may not experience any symptoms at all and go on to have healthy pregnancies. However even if fibroids are small and symptom free, steps should be taken to prevent further growth and reduce risk of new fibroid formation.

Treatment

Medications

Danazol
This drug helps to reduce the size of the fibroid and is often prescribed prior to surgery. This should not be taken if trying to conceive as it can cause serious harm to an unborn baby.

GnRH agonists
These drugs commence a medical induced menopause and are therefore also not suitable if wanting to conceive

Surgery
Surgery is one of the only medical options available and drugs are generally only prescribed prior to surgery.

Myomectomy
The aim of a myomectomy is to remove existing fibroids. However it won't stop new fibroids growing back. This is the only surgical option for women still wanting to conceive.

Hysterectomy
Hysterectomy is the complete removal of the uterus. For obvious reasons, this is not an option for women wishing to conceive.

Uterine fibroid embolization
This procedure helps to shrink or completely destroy existing fibroids however it can throw the body into early menopause and cause infertility. Therefore this is not a suitable option for those wanting to conceive.

Herbal support

Ginger (Zingiber officinalis)
Ginger is excellent for supporting circulation to the uterus as well as reducing inflammation. It's also a great anti-nausea for morning sickness in the early stages of pregnancy.

Recommended dose – 500 – 1000mg per day or fresh ginger can be grated and used to make herbal tea.

Raspberry leaf
Raspberry leaf helps to tone the uterine muscles as well as helping to normalise menstrual blood flow. It also possesses astringent properties, which can be beneficial for supporting the contraction of fibroids and reducing excessive bleeding.

Recommended dose – 400 – 800mg 3 x per day or 2 – 4 cups of raspberry leaf tea per day

Nutritional support

Iron
Iron deficiency is relatively common in women with fibroids due to the regular heavy bleeding. Ensure a healthy intake of iron rich foods and have your iron levels checked by your Health Care Professional to see if supplementation is required

Recommended dose – 5 – 24mg per day

Food sources – Oysters, beef, turkey, chicken, pork, fish, soybeans, lentils, kidney beans, spinach, tofu

Milk thistle

Milk thistle is a gentle liver tonic to support clearance of excess estrogen. It also provide mild anti-inflammatory action

Recommended dose – 10,000 – 15,000mg
2-3 times per day

Diet

DIET SHOULD FOCUS ON:
- ✓ Whole foods
- ✓ Focus on vegetables and vegetable based protein sources
- ✓ Limit red meat, which can exacerbate inflammation and focus on white meat or vegetarian iron sources
- ✓ Increase fibre to support estrogen clearance eg.
- ✓ Dark green leafy vegetables
- ✓ Broccoli
- ✓ Quinoa
- ✓ Chia seeds
- ✓ Flaxseeds
- ✓ Quinoa
- ✓ Beans and legumes
- ✓ Wholegrains such as brown rice, spelt, millet, oats, rye, barley and buckwheat

SOME FOODS MAY CONTRIBUTE TO ESTROGEN EXCESS, SO YOU SHOULD AVOID:
- ✓ Processed, refined white grains
- ✓ Processed/junk foods
- ✓ Caffeine
- ✓ Alcohol
- ✓ Saturated/trans fats

The 90 day fertility diet at the end of this book is ideal for those with fibroids.

Exercise

Exercise helps to stimulate healthy circulation to prevent stagnation and help alleviate congestion. Aim to exercise for around 30 minutes 5 times per week. Particularly core exercises focusing on the uterine region can be beneficial such as belly dancing, Pilates and yoga or even grab yourself an old fashioned hula hoop!

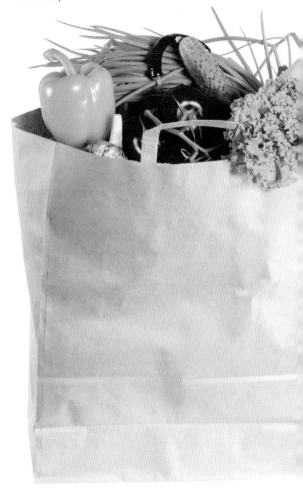

Enhancing your overall fertility

WOMEN

Key Nutrients

Deficiency of essential micronutrients, are associated with significant reproductive risks ranging from infertility to impaired fetal development and long term disease predisposition in the infant. The period just prior to conception plays a significant role in determining not only fertilization potential but also risk of miscarriage and fetal development issues, including congenital abnormalities, disrupted fetal growth, premature birth and complications for the mother.

Here, I have outlined the most important nutrients to help improve fertility and conception as well as supporting the progression of a healthy pregnancy. However, when supplementing I do recommend taking these nutrients either within, or in combination with, a good quality multivitamin and a healthy dietary intake. The recommended doses are to be used only as a guide, your Health Care Professional may prescribe higher levels if deficiency has been diagnosed.

Folate

Folate, also known as vitamin B9, is necessary to maintain healthy hormone balance and ovarian function, it also plays a critical in the development of DNA and is therefore essential to embryo development.

Homocysteine is a marker of inflammation in the body and can impact fertility and pregnancy. High homocysteine levels are common in people with high stress, high cholesterol or other disease states. High homocysteine levels are also more common in women with Polycystic Ovarian Syndrome (PCOS).

Some women with PCOS may be prescribed insulin sensitisers such as Metformin, to help improve ovulation function. This can be effective in many women, however these drugs also deplete folate levels, therefore a high folate diet and supplementation is essential for these women particularly. This is also the case for women losing weight. Although weight loss (to reach a healthy BMI) is highly beneficial to fertility and conception, homocysteine levels rise during this period and an adequate supply of folate becomes even more important.

Women taking folate supplements have been found to have higher quality eggs and a higher level of maturity in their eggs than women who don't supplement. Folate is also vital for early embryo development. The amount of folate present in the egg and sperm at the time of fertilization, impacts the development of the embryo.

When taking folate supplements, it's important to be aware of the difference between folate and folic acid. Folate is the natural nutrient used by the body and folic acid is a synthetic supplemental source of folate. A common genetic polymorphism, found in up to 50% of women, impairs the body's ability to convert synthetic folic acid into natural folate. This polymorphism significantly impacts folate levels, which subsequently affects hormone function, ovarian function, ovulation, embryo development as well as risk of miscarriage, birth defects and your ability to conceive. It's best to look for a supplement providing folate in the form of calcium folinate or folinic acid. These forms of supplemental folate do not pose the same metabolic issues and have been clinically proven to increase folate levels more effectively than folic acid.

Recommended therapeutic dose – 500mg of calcium folinate/folinic acid per day

Food sources – Asparagus, brussel sprouts, romaine lettuce, beans, soy beans, lentils, peas, sweet potato, broccoli, great leafy vegetables, sprouts, oranges, oatmeal, wheat germ

Choline

Choline is an essential nutrient involved in the development, structure and function of every cell in our body. During pregnancy it is particularly essential alongside folate for the development of the neural tube, which occurs very early on in pregnancy, before you may even be aware you're pregnant. Choline also helps support healthy brain development, supports healthy growth of the placenta as well as reducing the risk of miscarriage.

"The importance of choline cannot be overstated as we continue to unravel the role it plays in human health and development" - Gerald Weissmann MD, Editor-in-Chief FASEB Journal.

Research shows that 90% of women aren't reaching their recommended adequate intake of this important nutrient so supplementation during the conception period is advised. This is largely due to the fact that choline is one of the 'newest' nutrients, only added to the list of required human nutrients in 1998. It was previously believed that our bodies produced enough choline from other nutrients however recent data shows that dietary intake is essential to meet the body's demand, especially during the important months of conception, pregnancy and breastfeeding.

Recommended therapeutic dose – 400mg – 500mg of choline per day

Food sources – lecithin granules, eggs, beef, salmon, chicken, baked beans, kidney beans, lentils, brussel sprouts, broccoli, spinach, cauliflower, wheatgerm, oats and milk.

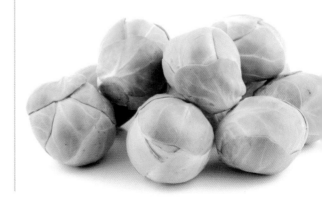

Vitamin B12

Vitamin B12 works alongside folate in the reduction of homocysteine and inflammation as well as the development of DNA. Lack of this important nutrient can impact fertility and ability to conceive as well as affecting the progression of a healthy pregnancy. Vitamin B12 helps support regular ovulation and aids in the healthy development of the endometrium lining to enable successful fertilization. Deficiency of this essential nutrient can cause infertility.

The great thing about vitamin B12 is that deficiency can be quickly and easily rectified through a healthy intake of vitamin 12 rich foods and supplementation. When supplementing either folate or vitamin B12, it's best to take these important nutrients together in a similar dose. This is not only due to their unique combined action but also because high folate levels can mask vitamin B12 deficiency. Lack of this critical nutrient during pregnancy can also impact the long-term health of the child.

Recommended therapeutic dose – 500mg per day

Food sources – Beef, crab, clams, oysters, lamb, tuna, trout, salmon, sardines, veal, milk, yoghurt, cheese, eggs

Vitamin B6

Vitamin B6 is required for hormone production and regulation. Therapeutic doses of vitamin B6 are commonly used in the treatment of hormonal conditions including PMT, PMS, menstrual regulation and morning sickness of pregnancy. Women are more likely to be deficient in vitamin B6 than men, although the reason for this is unknown it may be due to its role in hormone regulation. Vitamin B6 is also more common in women taking the Pill with research showing that up to 40% of women using this form of contraception, have biochemical evidence of deficiency.

Due to its hormone balancing properties, research shows that vitamin B6 may have a positive impact on fertility and the progression of a healthy pregnancy.

Deficiency is directly impacted by the amount of processed foods consumed. Those following a whole food diet (as per the 90-day fertility diet) are significantly less likely to be deficient in vitamin B6. However even healthy diets struggle to reach a therapeutic level of vitamin B6, therefore supplementation can be beneficial.

Recommended therapeutic dose – 50 – 100mg per day (more may be prescribed by your Health Care Professional however this does should not be exceeded unless under medical supervision)

Food sources – Fish, chicken, veal, pork, beef, eggs, lentils, split peas, kidney beans, peanuts, walnuts, sunflower seeds, avocado, bananas, brussel sprouts, sweet potato, carrots, peas, whole grains

Vitamin D

Vitamin D plays a vital role in fertility due to its role in the production and regulation of sex hormones. Vitamin D deficiency is extremely common affecting around 80% of women and has been found to be more common in women visiting fertility clinics. In a study from Yale University School of Medicine it was found that only 7% of infertile women, had normal levels of vitamin D.

A recent review of current data relating to the impact of vitamin D deficiency on fertility showed that healthy vitamin D levels improve fertility and ability to conceive and carry a healthy pregnancy. Healthy vitamin D levels are associated with higher rates of successful pregnancy in those undergoing

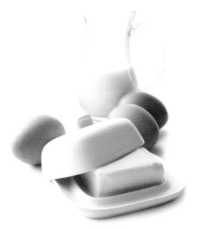

IVF treatment. Studies suggest that this may be due to a role in improving implantation and immune balance to support acceptance of the embryo. Supplementation was also found to be effective in improving fertility issues associated with Polycystic Ovarian Syndrome (PCOS). Another study showed that women with PCOS have been found to have lower levels of vitamin D than healthy, fertile women. Vitamin D deficiency may also help to protect against endometriosis.

> Recommended therapeutic dose – 1000IU per day
>
> Food sources – There are limited food sources of vitamin D, these include milk, butter, salmon, tuna, cod liver oil, herring liver oil, prawns, egg yolk
>
> The most potent natural source is sun exposure.

Iron

Iron works in combination with folate and vitamin B12 in the development of DNA and is therefore essential to healthy fetal development. Severe iron deficiency is associated with reduced fertility and conception rates and negatively impacts the progression of a healthy pregnancy.

However, it's important to remember that iron is a heavy metal. It is stored in our fat reserves and our body has no means by which to excrete excess. Therefore, supplementation should be monitored and never exceed the recommended dose unless under medical supervision. Australian, New Zealand, US and Canadian guidelines recommend an intake of 18mg prior to conception increasing to 27mg during pregnancy, with an upper safe limit of 45mg. Varying standards exist across the globe with the World Health Organization recommending maximal supplementation of 60mg for a maximum 6 months of pregnancy whereas the UK don't recommend any supplementation unless anaemia has been diagnosed and intake both prior to and during pregnancy is recommended to be 14.8mg.

There are varying forms of iron supplements, the most common being ferrous sulphate, ferrous fumarate and iron amino acid chelate. Ferrous sulphate is the cheapest form of iron but also the least well absorbed and most likely to cause gastric disturbance and constipation. Ferrous fumarate is a more natural source with slightly better absorption and reduced side effects, however the best form of iron supplement to look for is an iron amino acid chelate. Chelated minerals are more easily absorbed by the body resulting in a better uptake into cells and greatly reduced incidence of side effects.

For these reasons, it's good to have your iron levels checked prior to conception, boost your intake of iron rich foods and supplement with a good quality multivitamin including an iron amino acid chelate, not exceeding the recommended dose.

Food sources

There are 2 different forms of iron, heme iron from meat sources and non-heme iron from vegetarian sources. Heme sources are more quickly and easily absorbed than non-heme sources, however metabolism of non-heme sources increases when iron levels are low. Therefore vegetarians can get enough iron from their diet so long as the include plenty of vegetarian iron sources.

HEME IRON
Oysters, Beef, Turkey, Chicken, Pork, Fish

NON-HEME IRON
Soybeans, lentils, kidney beans, molasses, spinach, tofu

Recommended therapeutic dose – 24mg per day

Iodine
Iodine is used by the body to produce the thyroid hormones triiodothyronine (T3) and thyroxine (T4). Healthy thyroid function is essential for fertility, conception and healthy fetal development. If the thyroid does not have sufficient iodine to produce adequate thyroid hormones this can cause ovulatory problems and inability to ovulate, which can result in infertility.

Iodine during pregnancy is vital for healthy brain and nervous system development. Lack of iodine during pregnancy is the most common cause of preventable mental retardation worldwide. In severe cases, deficiency of this essential nutrient can also cause cretinism; symptoms include severely stunted physical and mental growth. Iodine deficiency is a common worldwide health problem. The average diet is very low in iodine and therefore the World Health Organisation recommend supplementation during pregnancy. Most of the world's iodine in found in the ocean, this is why seaweed is one of your best sources of dietary iodine. Women who are currently taking thyroid medication or who have a pre-existing condition should consult their Health Care Professional before taking iodine supplements.

Recommended therapeutic dose – 150 - 250mcg per day

Food sources – Seaweed and other sea vegetables, fish, shellfish, yoghurt, cow's milk, strawberries, eggs, mozzarella cheese

Zinc
As the egg reaches maturation and prepares to be released during ovulation, major biochemical changes take place to prepare the egg for potential fertilization. This process is critically dependent on zinc. Zinc levels within the egg have been shown to increase by 30 – 50% during this time and overall zinc levels within the body have a significant effect on the egg maturation process impacting fertilization and embryo development. Acute zinc deficiency has been found to cause profound defects during this period, which can prevent ovulation and fertilization. A clinical trial showed that a zinc deficient diet 3 – 5 days before ovulation dramatically disrupted the maturation process. Ovulation rates remained similar in the acutely zinc deficient group however the zinc deficient diet significantly reduced fertilization rate by almost 50% and in those that were fertilised the embryos were less competent. If pregnancy does occur, continued zinc deficiency can lead to significant developmental issues. Zinc also supports the absorption of folate.

Recommended therapeutic dose – 15 – 40mg per day

Food sources – Oysters, shellfish, canned fish, red meat, pork, hard cheese, nuts, pulses, wholegrain

Antioxidants

Antioxidants help protect the body, and in the case of fertility the precious developing egg, from free radical damage. Free radicals are basically damaged cells, which are described as 'free' because they are missing a critical molecule which spurs them to seek out other molecules to pair with. Unfortunately when these free radicals pair with another healthy cell, they damage that cell, often injuring the DNA, which can lead to development of disease or simply accelerate the aging process. The simple process of living creates a small amount of free radicals, which increases as we age. Factors such as smoking, alcohol, exposure to toxins, stress and poor diet increase the amount of free radicals our body produces.

Antioxidants assist by pairing with these free radicals and deeming them harmless. This stops them from pairing with, and damaging, other healthy cells.

GOOD NUTRITIONAL
ANTIOXIDANTS INCLUDE:

✓ Betacarotene
✓ Vitamin C
✓ Vitamin E
✓ Co enzyme Q10

Herbs

Herbs can be a wonderfully supportive addition to fertility treatment and below I've outlined some of my favourite nourishing and nurturing herbs. However, herbs that play a role in hormone regulation should only be used on the advice of a Health Care Professional who can provide a complete prescription tailored to your individual needs. Self-prescribing these herbs without supervision may be harmful. For this reason I have not suggested a recommended dose for these herbs.

Hormone Balance

Vitex-agnus castus (Chaste Tree Berry)

This well-known herb has a strong history of traditional use and is known as the Queen of women's conditions. Vitex has been used for centuries in the treatment of various gynaecological conditions. Over the past 50 years it has been adopted by the mainstream European medical profession and in Germany it is recognised by the German Commission for the treatment of menstrual irregularities and PMS and is commonly prescribed by gynaecologists and GP's.

Vitex helps support the production of progesterone, yet contains no actual hormones itself. Vitex helps correct hormonal imbalance at the source by exerting its effect on the hypothalamic-pituitary-ovarian axis (hormonal feedback loop). For this reason unlike synthetic progesterone, Vitex can take 3 to 12 cycles to exert its full benefit.

Vitex is effective in relieving symptoms of PMS and is beneficial to help regulate the menstrual cycle. Vitex is particularly useful for those suffering amenorrhoea (lack of menstruation), low progesterone levels, high relative estrogen levels or luteal phase defects. This powerful women's herb supports the secretion of luteinising hormone, which in turn increases progesterone. Progesterone is vital for healthy ovulation a healthy luteal phase, both of which are essential for conception to occur.

As explained in more depth in chapter 'The Basics', luteal phase is the time after ovulation and before your next period, when the uterine lining thickens to prepare for a potential pregnancy. If this phase is too short, (less than 12 – 14 days) the lining does not have adequate time to prepare and an egg is not able to successfully implant. Vitex can assist in lengthening this time frame to help encourage healthy thickening of the uterine lining to support successful implantation.

Vitex has also been traditionally used in cases of threatened miscarriage, however it should only be used for this action under medical supervision.

Shatavari

I love the history of this herb. Shatavari has been used for centuries in Indian Ayurvedic practice and the name translates to "she who possess a hundred husbands". The name is presumed to have originated from its extensive use as a reproductive and fertility tonic. Shatavari has a widespread action on the reproductive system. This wonderful women's tonic is excellent for those with high stress levels, acting as a nervous system tonic to help reduce stress levels as well as helping to regulate hormone balance and support regular menstruation and ovulation. Shatavari also provides immune support, helping to balance the immune system to encourage embryo acceptance as well as supporting the body's mucous membranes, which can be particularly useful for women with low cervical mucus. Traditionally, shatavari has

been prescribed in cases of threatened miscarriage however this should only be administered on the advice of a Health Care Professional.

Paeonia lactiflora (Peony)

Peony is a popular Chinese herb commonly prescribed for a range of reproductive conditions including PMS, polycystic ovarian syndrome (PCOS), anovulation, endometriosis, androgen excess and infertility. Peony is commonly prescribed in combination with other supportive herbs including liquorice and dong quai because studies have shown it performs better within a synergistic combination. Studies indicate that Peony exerts its hormonal action by stimulating aromatase enzyme activity. Aromatase is found throughout the body particularly in the ovaries, the liver and fatty tissue where it plays an important role in hormone production and ovulation. Low aromatase activity can lead to erratic ovulation and can interfere with estrogen levels. Peony assists in normalising hormonal balance, supporting progesterone production and reducing androgen levels.

Dong Quai (Angelica sinensis)

Chinese medicine refers to dong quai as a female tonic and blood tonic. It's a supportive, nourishing herb, which can be beneficial for women experiencing lack of energy after periods, irregular or absent periods and light or pale menstrual flow. It can also be useful for those wanting to stimulate a regular cycle following the cessation of the Pill as well as having a strengthening effect on the uterus. However, although Dong quai is a wonderful herb to help support fertility it should be used with caution. It should not be used in women with heavy menstrual bleeding or blood thinning medications and should be discontinued at least 2 weeks prior to any surgical procedures. It should also not be used during pregnancy or if there is the possibility of pregnancy. Therefore I recommend consulting a qualified natural health practitioner before embarking on treatment.

Nourishing/Nervous system tonics

Nettle
Nettle is a great nourishing herb, particularly beneficial for those who experience heavy menstrual bleeding and/or low iron levels. Taken in either capsules as a herbal tea, nettles are high in iron and vitamin C whilst also supporting liver function.

Recommended dose – 2000 – 4000mg
3 times per day

Raspberry leaf
Raspberry leaf is well known for its role in supporting uterine tone in the lead up to delivery, however this unique pregnancy herb can also be beneficial to support uterine tone and general health of the uterus prior to conception. It's also a good source of vitamin A, B complex, vitamin C, vitamin C, iron, calcium, potassium and silica. Raspberry leaf should only be used prior to conception and in the third trimester of pregnancy under advisement of your health care professional.

Recommended dose - 400mg 3 times a day
or 2 – 3 cups of raspberry leaf tea per day

MACA root (Lepidium meyenii)
MACA is extremely high in natural nutrients providing over 30 minerals and 60 nutrients. For this reason, it has a long history of traditional use as tonic for energy virility, libido and fertility. Clinical studies have confirmed its traditional use with subjects reporting increased sexual desire. MACA is a beneficial addition to the diet of those with low energy, physical or mental exhaustion.

Recommended dose – 1500 – 3000mg
or 1 heaped tsp of MACA powder per day

Oats
Oats are one of my favourite herbs. I find them particularly indicated as a tonic to support the nervous system and generally nourish the body to prepare for pregnancy. Oats are particularly beneficial for those suffering from stress and exhaustion.

Recommended dose – 1000 – 4000mg
3 times per day

Withania somnifera/Indian ginseng
With use dating back to 6000BC, Withania is one of our oldest 'folk' medicines, traditionally used as a tonic for the reproductive system, nervous system and for general health. Withania supports both stress reduction and fertility by helping to reduce cortisol levels, which are found to be high in stressed individuals. High cortisol levels can greatly impact fertility and overall general health. With no direct action on the hormonal system, Withania is used to support both male and female fertility.

Recommended dose – 3000mg – 9000mg
per day

Detoxification/ Anti-inflammatory

Milk Thistle/St Mary's Thistle (Silymarin/Silybum marinanum)

An overloaded or low functioning liver impairs the body's ability to remove toxins from the body as well as affecting hormone production. Therefore it's important for both males and females to ensure healthy liver function to support fertility and conception. During pregnancy there is a greater demand on the liver as it processes the additional hormones circulating in your system so ensuring healthy liver function prior to conception can also support the progression of a healthy pregnancy. Milk thistle is one of the most well-known and widely used liver tonics, acting as a protectant as well as supporting the body's detoxification pathways. Milk thistle also provides antioxidant and anti-inflammatory activity as well as supporting healthy immune function. Numerous clinical studies have confirmed Milk thistles long history of traditional use.

> Recommended dose – 10,000 – 15,000mg
> 2-3 times per day

Turmeric

Turmeric is particularly useful in supporting detoxification pathways in the liver whilst also providing antioxidant and anti-inflammatory action. Clinical studies confirm its beneficial role in supporting detoxification, particularly in reducing the impact of exposure to heavy metals including arsenic, cadmium, chromium, copper, lead and mercury on the liver, all of which can impact fertility, conception and the progression of a healthy pregnancy. This can be especially useful for those previously or currently exposed to these toxins. Turmerics strong antioxidant action also protects liver cells against all forms of oxidative stress.

> Recommended dose – 400 – 600mg
> 3 times per day

Calendula

Calendula is probably more commonly known for its external use in creams for its antiseptic and wound healing properties. However used internally Calendula helps to improve lymphatic drainage and circulation, which is particularly beneficial for those suffering fluid retention and to help reduce the pelvic congestion of endometriosis. Calendula also helps to regulate excessive menstrual bleeding as well as reducing inflammation and is therefore beneficial for those suffering heavy periods or clotting. It also exerts a gentle balancing action on the immune system.

> Recommended dose – 1000 – 4000g dried
> flowers 3 times per day

Ginger

Ginger is a wonderful warming, comforting herb. It helps promote circulation as well as providing anti-inflammatory activity. Ginger is particularly indicated in those suffering endometriosis and painful periods. Ginger is also a wonderful herb to keep in your cupboard during pregnancy for its proven relief against morning sickness.

> Recommended dose – 500 – 1000mg per day
> or fresh ginger can be grated and used to make
> an herbal tea.

Exercise

Too much exercise will negatively impact fertility. Women participating in regular high intensity, strenuous exercise show increased cortisol levels (as found in those with high stress levels) and reduced thyroid hormones. Both of these factors can reduce fertility as well as affecting hormone balance. High impact training can reduce the body's ability to produce progesterone, which is critical for ovulation. Extremely athletic women also have greatly reduced levels of body fat. Low body fat has a direct impact on estrogen production, reducing estrogen levels, which can lead to irregular or complete loss of the menstrual cycle as well as irregular is absence of ovulation.

However, before you throw out your trainers, at the other extreme, very little exercise will also negatively impact your ability to conceive. Just as women with very little body fat, may suffer from reduced estrogen production, those with excess body fat may experience increased estrogen production. This can have the same effect on the menstrual cycle, causing irregular or loss of periods as well as irregular or lack of ovulation. Also, just as regular strenuous activity can increase cortisol levels, lack of exercise can also increase cortisol levels. Regular moderate exercise aids the body's natural stress response, improving our ability to deal with stress as well as helping to reduce cortisol levels.

So what is the 'right amount' of exercise? Although there is no finite definition of exactly how many hours and how much intensity is optimal for each individual, most specialists agree that 30 minutes of activity 3 – 4 times per week is a great step towards boosting fertility. For those who already participate in slightly more than this, that's likely to be fine, however if you are exceeding 7 hours per week it would be wise to consider cutting back. If you're concerned whether you're over or under doing it, it's best to speak with your Health Care Professional about the level they suggest would be best for you.

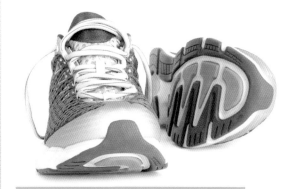

HEALTHY EXERCISE ACTIVITIES INCLUDE:
- ✓ brisk walking
- ✓ jogging
- ✓ leisurely bike riding
- ✓ yoga
- ✓ light aerobics
- ✓ dancing

ACTIVITIES TO AVOID INCLUDE:
- ✓ marathon running/training
- ✓ daily 'boot camp'
- ✓ daily strenuous sports
- ✓ heavy weight lifting
- ✓ any exercise over an hour in duration more than 7 times per week

Stress

Stress is not a healthy state for the body to be in. Our body recognises this, by actively reducing our ability to conceive in times of extreme stress. Stress sends us into 'fight or flight' mode, releasing the stress hormones, adrenaline and cortisol, to prime the body ready for attack or retreat. This stress hormone release is extremely valuable and effective when a tiger is bounding towards us and we need immediate energy to either grapple with the beast or swiftly run away. However in today's society, our stressors aren't generally as acute. Work pressure or family difficulties can elicit the same response, however with no immediate end in sight our body can remain in this hyper-vigilant state. This leaves us with continuing high levels of stress hormones in our system, which is in itself harmful to the body as well as reducing our ability to produce reproductive hormones necessary for conception. Chronic stress has become such a common factor in infertility that it has gained its own name 'Stress Induced Reproductive Dysfunction.' High stress can also exacerbate complications of infertility stemming from other causes as well as reducing effectiveness of IVF treatment.

So what can you do?

Stress is a natural part of our daily life and healthy levels can actually be productive, but when stress levels exceed our coping mechanisms and begin to negatively impact our health some strategies need to be implemented to help combat this.

Reduce stressors

This one sounds simple but may be hard to implement. The main thing is to prioritise. What stressors can you realistically reduce or delete from your life? Can you change jobs? Reduce responsibilities? Get help at home?

Getting enough sleep

Getting enough good quality sleep can greatly improve our ability to deal with stress, improve mood and improve fertility. Women who have difficulty sleeping or work night shift are more likely to suffer not only higher stress levels but more hormonal imbalance. Sleep affects vital reproductive hormones including estrogen, progesterone, luteinising hormone and follicle stimulating hormone as well as leptin. Leptin is a hormone specifically linked to sleep, as healthy amounts are only produced when we're achieving adequate sleep. Inability to produce healthy levels of leptin directly impacts they body's ability to ovulate.

Although it may sound simple, many people aren't achieving the 8 hour per day goal. And this doesn't mean, 2 hours dosing in front of the TV or iPad, or lying awake running over your 'to do' list for the next day. Ideally an hour before bed should be your 'wind down' time, taking your mind off stressors of the day and preparing the body for a restful sleep. This will help enable your body to more quickly reach REM (rapid eye movement) sleep. Frequent waking, or 'light' sleeping means your body is not properly entering this deep sleep phase. To support healthy sleep patterns it's important to reduce caffeine intake, particularly prior to bed, increase 'wind down' time before bed, sleep in a darkened room and reduce amount of 'screen time' before bed.

Regular moderate exercise

As outlined above

Meditation and/or yoga

Yoga and meditation can help reduce stress by focusing on the inner body, which helps to reduce your focus on external pressures and stressors. In a study of women who had been trying to conceive for 1 – 2 years, showed that those who participated in mind-body therapy had a 42% incidence of spontaneous conception compared to only 11 – 20% for those who didn't participate.

Acupuncture

IVF clinics are now regularly aligned with acupuncture clinics with patients finding it beneficial to help regulate cycles, reduce stress and improve overall fertility.

Kinesiology/Reflexology

I myself found Kinesiology to be very useful in my quest to fall pregnant and I recommend utilising alternative health practitioners such as this to help improve your fertility as well as reducing the stress that often goes hand in hand with fertility issues. Look for a practitioner who specialises in fertility issues or ask friends or family who may be able to refer you to a practitioner they trust.

Natural calming herbs

Chamomile tea has long been recognised for its therapeutic relaxing properties and can be a great addition to a healthy diet. Other useful herbs include passionflower, withania, lemon balm as well as valerian and zizyphus for a stronger sedating action to help promote restful sleep. Most of these herbs can be sourced easily in the form of teas or over the counter natural sleep tablets and preparations. For those suffering extreme chronic stress or sleep disturbance, it would be valuable to seek assistance from a qualified natural health practitioner who can tailor a nutritional and herbal program to best suit your needs.

Talk

If writing isn't enough to reduce your stress levels, talking can help. Whether this is to a trusted friend or ideally a qualified counsellor, allowing others to support you in a situation which is overwhelming can greatly reduce stress levels and significantly improve ongoing coping mechanisms.

Vitamins and minerals

Chronic stress can deplete the body of essential nutrients, which in turn reduce our ability to cope with stress. The most important nutrients to consider during times of stress include all the B complex vitamins, vitamin D and magnesium.

Write a journal or keep a notebook

We often keep all our stressors bottled up in our head. Spinning them around and around until they seem insurmountable! Simply writing your stressors or 'to do' list down on paper helps to break the cycle and can give you a clearer picture of the tasks that need your attention and the ones that can be temporarily set aside.

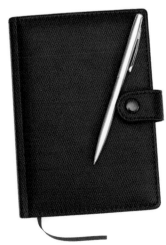

IMPROVING EGG QUALITY

Healthy eggs are vital for a healthy conception. They ultimately decide whether fertilisation and implantation occur and whether the pregnancy will be viable.

We hear and talk a lot about poor egg quality greatly impacting our ability to conceive. But what exactly is 'poor egg quality'?

In actual fact there is no scientific measure of egg quality and what constitutes good or poor, but rather this is simply a subjective measure and opinion. It is true that the quality of our eggs reduce as we age and that this impacts our ability to conceive, however there are things we can do to nurture our eggs through the maturation process to give them the best chance possible. We may not have control over our biological clock but we do have control over the environment and nutrient status in which our eggs develop.

The 90 day life cycle of the egg

Female babies are born are born with approximately 1 million potential eggs. These eggs slowly die off, reaching around 300,000 – 400,000 at puberty. During the reproductive years, women will release around 350 – 450 of these eggs during ovulation. Each potential egg (or follicle) lies dormant in the ovaries until it receives the signal go grow and mature, a process called folliculogenesis. Around a hundred follicles begin this process however only one will become the dominant follicle and produce fully developed egg, which is then released at ovulation. Although it has been long believed that females were born with all the eggs they would ever have, which slowly die off over time until reaching menopause, science is an evolving field and new research suggests that women may actually have the ability to produce more eggs during her reproductive years. Although yet to be confirmed, this theory which has already been proven in animal studies, gives hope that we can have an even greater influence over the health of our eggs and our fertility than ever before.

This includes the amount of blood flow, amount of oxygen available, the woman's nutritional status, hormonal balance and stress levels. By the time the menstrual cycle commences around 3 – 30 follicles remain, which will then eventuate in one dominant follicle (or in rarer cases multiple dominant follicles) producing one mature egg for release at ovulation. So here's what you can do to support healthy follicle development in the 'survival of the fittest' race to produce one spectacularly healthy egg!

Blood flow

Improving blood flow to the ovaries helps carry oxygen and important nutrients to where they are most needed.

SUPPORT HEALTHY BLOOD FLOW BY:
Ensuring adequate hydration
Lack of hydration can increase the thickness of the blood, reducing the ability to easily flow around the body. Ideally, you should aim for 2 litres/8 glasses of water per day.

Exercise

As discussed earlier, healthy levels of activity can positively influence fertility. One of the ways in which it achieves this is by improving blood flow. The more we move, the more our blood is pumped around our body, transporting vital nutrients.

Herbal supplements

To complement the above practices you may wish to combine some simple herbal treatments to further stimulate blood flow. Ginkgo biloba and ginger are excellent herbs for supporting healthy blood flow.

Nutrition

What you eat during these important 90 days can positively or negatively influence your egg health.

IT'S IMPORTANT TO INCREASE YOUR INTAKE OF:

✓ fresh, organic fruits and vegetables
✓ whole grains
✓ nuts and seeds
✓ oily fish
✓ organic meats

AND DECREASE YOUR INTAKE OF:

✓ caffeine
✓ alcohol
✓ soft drinks
✓ refined sugar
✓ processed foods
✓ non-organic meats
✓ genetically modified foods

The 90 day fertility diet, found at the end of this book, has been specifically designed to help optimise the health of your eggs during this critical window.

Supplements

If only we still all sourced our fruits and vegetables from the veggie patch in the backyard and our meat came from the free roaming cattle in the paddock. Unfortunately today, most of our food purchases are made from supermarket shelves where little is known about their origin or the steps that it's taken to reach these shelves. A healthy supply of nutrients is so important during this crucial phase that it's difficult to rely on diet alone to ensure adequate supply. A good prenatal multivitamin should never be a replacement for a healthy diet, however it can provide a healthy baseline of essential nutrients to compliment a balanced diet. I see a good multivitamin as an 'insurance policy' helping to ensure a healthy balance of essential nutrients regardless of fluctuations in daily dietary intake. You may also wish to include a good antioxidant such as co enzyme Q10 to further support egg health.

Stress

Stress has a negative impact on overall fertility as well as egg health specifically. Stress produces excess cortisol, which can interfere with hormone production during the egg cycle and can also increase the production of free radicals. Following the stress reducing guidelines outlined in this book (page 56) will help in improving overall fertility as well as egg health. In ideal conditions, the monthly shedding and rebuilding of the uterine lining provides the perfect environment for implantation and the progression of a healthy pregnancy.

UTERINE HEALTH

However, for some women, even with healthy eggs, the uterine environment may not be conducive to implantation and the egg 'just won't stick'. These have women have difficulty holding a pregnancy and are prone to early miscarriage.

CONDITIONS AFFECTING UTERINE HEALTH:
✓ Uterine fibroids
✓ Endometriosis
✓ PCOS
✓ Uterine scarring, resulting from previous abortion, dilation and curette (D&C), IUD, caesarean, abdominal or uterine surgery or pelvic inflammatory disease (PID)

As discussed in more detail on page 61, depending on their severity, these conditions can be successfully treated to improve uterine health and enable successful implantation and maintenance of a healthy pregnancy.

Other factors affecting uterine health

Sedentary lifestyle

Lack of activity and exercise decreases blood flow to the reproductive organs including the uterus. Decreased blood flow means less nutrients being carried to the uterus and more stagnation and congestion. A sedentary lifestyle can also impact the health of the muscular tissue of the uterus, weakening uterine strength.

Hormonal imbalance

Any factors affecting hormonal balance can negatively impact uterine health. Irregular menstruation, short, long, unusually light or heavy cycles can affect the body's ability to properly shed the endometrium. The endometrium relies on hormonal cues to adequately shed and rebuild a healthy lining. Hormonal imbalance can lead to incomplete shedding or poor rebuilding of the uterine lining, affecting its ability to house and nurture an embryo. Healthy estrogen levels are required to build a thick, healthy lining. Inadequate levels can lead to a thin lining which is not conducive to implantation. A uterine lining less than 8mm thick is considered inadequate.

"When the world says, 'Give up,'
Hope whispers, 'Try one more time.'"
~ Anonymous

Synthetic hormones

Although these medications can be valuable to act as a contraceptive or to improve fertility, long-term use of synthetic hormones such as the Pill has been shown to reduce the thickness and health of the uterine lining. Ideally taking a 3 – 6 month break from these medications can help nourish and support uterine health.

Improving
uterine health

Women with specific medical conditions affecting the health of their uterus will require specific treatment. However there are many things you can do to positively influence uterine health either in combination with these treatments or on their own for those with less specific uterine issues or who are just wanting to optimise uterine health.

Exercise

I talk a lot about activity and exercise throughout this book because it is so important for reproductive health. Regular gentle exercise such as walking, light jogging, or aerobics will help to stimulate blood flow to the uterus. To specifically address uterine health by focusing on the muscles surrounding the uterus, there are classes available for yoga and Pilates specifically focused on uterine tone and fertility enhancement.

Stress

Again a much mentioned topic in this book and for good reason. Stress reduces the body's ability to produce sex hormones required for reproduction, increases stress hormones,

reduces nutritional status as well as lessening important blood flow to the uterus.

Diet/Nutrition

Diet plays a key role in uterine health. Eating a healthy, balanced diet free from chemical contaminants helps nourish and support uterine health. The 90 day fertility diet outlined in this book helps support uterine health, egg health and overall fertility.

Supplements

OTHER KEY NUTRIENTS, WHICH CAN PLAY A SUPPORTIVE ROLE IN UTERINE HEALTH, INCLUDE:

✓ iron
✓ vitamin C
✓ vitamin E.

However as iron is a heavy metal, which is not easily excreted from the body, you should always have your iron levels checked before taking high dose supplements.

Herbs

The liver plays a major role in maintaining hormone balance as well as ridding the body of unwanted toxins, which can affect uterine health. A good liver tonic in combination with a healthy diet can be a useful addition. THESE INCLUDE:

✓ milk thistle
✓ turmeric

NOURISHING, BUILDING HERBS CAN ALSO BENEFIT UTERINE HEALTH, THESE INCLUDE:

✓ ginger
✓ raspberry leaf
✓ nettles

(refer to page 54 for a more detailed outline and dose recommendations for these herbs)

OVULATION ISSUES

Kick starting ovulation

Issues around ovulation, either irregular or anovulation, account for around 30 – 40% of infertility cases. The presentation can vary greatly. Some women may experience regular menstruation yet not be ovulating, for some women their cycles may vary in length each month making it hard to predict when ovulation is occurring. For most women, a good predictor of ovulatory dysfunction is when cycles are less than 21 days or longer than 36 days or in some cases women may have no menstrual bleeding at all.

This may be related to conditions such as PCOS or thyroid imbalance as discussed. However women may present with ovulation issues without the presence of any underlying disorders.

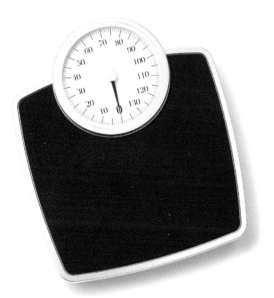

Diet

If very low or very high body weight is suspected to be the cause of ovulatory dysfunction, then diet and lifestyle modifications should be made before seeking medical treatment. Following the 90-day fertility diet as outlined in this book can help you reach and maintain a healthy body weight, which can stimulate natural ovulation. Those with very low body weight should increase the carbohydrate content of the diet by introducing larger portions of whole grains.

Exercise

As discussed previously, either excessive or lack of exercise can contribute to fertility issues. For guidelines on healthy exercise practices to boost your fertility, refer to page 55.

Lifestyle

Chronic, high level stress places the body in constant fight or flight mode. This triggers the release of adrenaline and cortisol, which can be beneficial stimulants in cases of acute stress but negatively impact health when they remain chronically high. For more information about how stress affects fertility and ways in which to overcome this, refer to page 56.

Nutritional support

Zinc
As discussed on page 50 zinc plays a role in supporting healthy ovulation and fertilization and may be beneficial where ovulatory dysfunction is present.

Vitamin B6
Vitamin B6 plays an important role in hormone production and regulation. As discussed on page 48 vitamin B6 can be beneficial to support healthy hormone balance to aid healthy ovulation. Supplementation of vitamin B6 can be particularly beneficial to help stimulate ovulation in those coming off hormonal contraception, as these medications can deplete the body of B6.

Herbal support
Vitex-agnus castus (Chaste Tree Berry)
Vitex is the most commonly prescribed herb for ovulatory dysfunction or anovulation. As discussed on page 51 it supports production of progesterone, which is vital for ovulation. It also helps regulate ovulation by supporting the lengthening of the luteal phase (the time from ovulation to the next menstrual period), which helps enable healthy fertilisation.

Medications

Clomiphene
Clomiphene (Clomid/Serophene) is commonly prescribed to help stimulate ovulation. It works by blocking estrogen receptors, which in turn stimulates the release of follicle stimulating hormone (FSH) and luteinising hormone (LH). These hormones are naturally released during the cycle to stimulate ovulation.

Clomiphene is taken for 5 days typically starting around day 3 – 5 of your cycle, or as recommended by your specialist. Ovulation will generally occur about 7 days after taking the last tablet. If the medication works and ovulation is stimulated yet pregnancy is not achieved, the dose can be repeated for 3 – 6 months. After this time, alternative treatment should be sought.

If clomiphene fails to stimulate ovulation the dose may be increased from 50 mg per day to 100mg then 150mg if necessary.

The use of clomiphene increases the chances of multiple births from 1% in the general population to 10%.

Injectable hormones
Depending on your presentation, your specialist may prescribe other injectable hormones to stimulate egg production.

The success rate of these medications stimulating ovulation is around 90% with pregnancy rates around 20 – 60%.

MEN

Men produce millions of sperm each day, in fact 1500 sperm are produced every second! There is much you can do to influence the health of these millions of sperm.

Key Nutrients

Zinc

Zinc is a trace mineral, meaning the body requires it in small amounts. However it's importance in male fertility cannot be underestimated. Zinc plays a pivitol role in sperm production, sperm health and testosterone production. Deficiency of this essential mineral is associated with decreased testosterone levels, low sperm count and low sperm motility. Studies have shown seminal plasma zinc levels to be significantly lower in infertile men and this may play a role in many cases of infertility of 'unknown cause'. Deficiency is associated with gonadal dysfunction, decreased testicular weight and shrinkage of seminiferous tubules, all of which greatly impact fertility.

Seminal plasma zinc levels are also strongly linked to sperm density and viability and supplementation has been shown to significantly improve sperm density, motility and improve conception and pregnancy outcomes. One study on patients with infertility related to low sperm count were found to have increased seminal zinc levels, improved sperm count and improved sperm health and motility after 4 months of zinc supplementation. 3 spontaneous pregnancies also occurred during the 4 months of the study.

Zinc is also involved in the transformation of testosterone into its active form, thereby boosting available testosterone in the system. A trial on patients with idiopathic infertility (infertility of unknown cause) of more than 5 years duration showed that supplementation with 24mg of zinc for 2 months dramatically increased testosterone levels in patients with previously low levels as well as significantly increasing sperm count from 8 million to 20 million/ml.

Recommended dose – 20 – 40mg per day

Carnitine

Carnitine is an amino acid involved in energy production. The highest concentrations of carnitine can be found in the epididymis (the tightly coiled tube within the testes which carries sperm) where it plays pivotal role in sperm motility, development and maturation. Infertile and subfertile men show lower levels of seminal carnitine than fertile men. Cartine has also been shown to provide antioxidant and anti-inflammatory activity, both of which further support sperm health. Studies have shown that increasing carnitine levels, through supplementation of 3g per day, not only increased sperm motility but also increased the number of viable sperm per ejaculate. Recent studies using 2-3g of carnitine per day showed increases in sperm motility, total number of sperm and increased ability to swim in a fast straight line as well as subsequent increases in pregnancy rates. Another recent study using 1g of carnitine per day showed significant improvements in sperm motility, number of 'A grade sperm' and number of normal shaped sperm.

Recommended dose – 1 – 3g per day.

Arginine

Arginine is another amino acid involved in sperm production as well as helping to improve blood flow. For this reason, arginine is commonly used in the treatment of erectile dysfunction.

The body can produce small amounts of arginine however in times of increased demand, dietary intake is necessary. Limited research has been done into arginine and fertility however studies have shown supplementation of 4g per day for 3 months – 6 months significantly improves sperm count and motility with subsequent improvements in pregnancy rates. Most improvements were found in men with sperm counts at or above 10 million/ml, below that, other confounding factors are believed to be at play and little benefit has been found. More research needs to be done on the mechanism of action of arginine in fertility and to confirm its effectiveness.

Recommended dose – 1 – 4g per day. Arginine can be taken as a single supplement or can be found as a component of protein and sports powders.

Co Enzyme Q10

Like carnitine, co enzyme Q10 is also involved in energy production as well as providing antioxidant activity. As coenzyme Q10 is so vital to energy production and to life itself, our body natural produces small amounts to support vital body functions. However our ability to produce coenzyme Q10 naturally decreases as we age and increase demand caused by stress, ageing and illness can further deplete our body's reserves. Therefore supplementation becomes more important as we age and the higher our stress levels. Co enzyme Q10 is found in significant amounts in seminal fluid. The amount of co enzyme Q10 present in seminal fluid is directly related to sperm count and motility. Studies involving supplementation with co enzyme Q10 have shown increases in sperm count and motility as well as increased pregnancy rates. A recent review of the many studies involving co enzyme Q10 concluded that co enzyme Q10 could provide effective treatment in many cases of unexplained infertility.

Recommended dose – 100 – 400mg per day

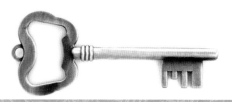

"Don't be discouraged. It's often the last key in the bunch that oprns the lock."

~ *Anonymous*

Vitamin B12

Vitamin B12 is essential to the production of DNA and RNA which are the building blocks upon which all cells are created. For this reason vitamin B12 is essential to fertility and conception in both males and females. In males, vitamin B12 is involved in sperm production and maturation. Studies have shown a 50 – 60% increase in sperm count in infertile men receiving 1500mg – 4000mg of vitamin B12 per day for 3 – 6 months. It should be noted that high dose vitamin B12 should be supplemented alongside the other members of the B vitamin family (ie. alongside a B complex supplement) to help maintain optimal balance.

Recommended dose – 500 – 1000mcg per day

Vitamin C

Vitamin C can be found in seminal plasma to help protect sperm and reduce oxidative damage. Low seminal plasma levels may contribute to infertility by increasing DNA damage. One study showed that by reducing vitamin C intake from 250mg per day to 5mg per day, seminal plasma levels dropped by 50 percent and sperm DNA damage increased by 91%. This shows that the amount of vitamin C found in seminal plasma is directly related to dietary intake. Being a water soluble vitamin, vitamin C is rapidly absorbed and can affect relatively immediate results. A study on infertile but otherwise healthy men supplemented with either 1000mg vitamin C, 200mg vitamin C or placebo showed a 140% increase in sperm count in the 1000mg group, a 114% increase in sperm count in the group receiving 200mg and no change in the placebo group. Both vitamin C supplemented groups also showed significant reduction in the number of 'sticky' sperm, or sperm stuck together, which also reduces fertility. However the most significant finding was that by the end of the 60 day trail, every participant in the vitamin C group had impregnated their partner, while no pregnancies occurred in the placebo group.

Cigarette smoking has been well documented to increase the body's demand for vitamin C, thus decreasing vitamin C levels. Therefore smokers have a much higher demand for vitamin C in order to maintain healthy seminal plasma levels.

Recommended dose – 2000 – 6000mg per day

Vitamin E

Vitamin E is well documented for its antioxidant properties. It has been shown to inhibit free radical damage in sperm helping to improve the number of healthy sperm as well as sperm motility and function. A randomised trial using 600mg of vitamin E per day showed improved ability of the sperm to penetrate the egg. Further studies confirm that vitamin E supplementation improves fertilization rates.

Recommended dose – 400 – 800IU per day

Selenium

Selenium is essential for sperm development. It is a component of selenoproteins. These proteins protect sperm against oxidative damage as well as being structural component of mature sperm. High concentrations of selenium are found in the testes and molecular studies show that the testes actively uptake and store selenium for this purpose. Lack of selenium results in poor sperm development and development of abnormal sperm. A recent study of male partners of infertile couples showed reduced selenium levels present in all male subjects.

Recommended dose – 100 – 200mcg per day

Antioxidants

Sperm are especially susceptible to the effects of oxidative stress, which is basically the stress caused by exposure to environmental factors. A recent review of antioxidant involvement in fertility demonstrated that many antioxidant nutrients including vitamin A, vitamin E, vitamin C, B complex, glutathione, co enzyme Q10, carnitine, zinc and selenium provide significant benefit in the treatment on male infertility. Antioxidants have also been shown to have a significant benefit in supporting the progression of a healthy embryo and pregnancy in men who've previously suffered recurrent embryo loss. A recent Cochrane review confirmed that men taking antioxidants had a statistically significant increase in pregnancy rates and the partner's ability to carry a healthy baby to term. Men undergoing IVF treatment whilst taking antioxidants showed a fourfold improvement in conceptions and live birth rates.

Herbs

Detoxification

Sperm is actually a one of the channels of detoxification. Therefore it's important to help ensure the main detox pathways via digestion and liver are working efficiently to rid the body of excess toxins and keep

sperm free and clear of any potential toxins. Studies show that fertility and semen quality can be greatly impacted by exposure to industrial lead, cadmium, zinc and copper. High levels in the blood stream have been shown to impact sperm density, total sperm count, sperm motility and viability as well as impacting testosterone balance. Even moderate exposure to lead and cadmium in particular can negatively impact semen quality and fertility without showing any significant impairment of reproductive function through standard testing.

Exposure to other heavy metals and modern chemicals such as PBC's, pesticides, chlorine and industrial pollutants can also impact sperm health. In fact the average male sperm quality and potency is believed to be up to half that of men 50 years ago, largely due the introduction of these chemicals into everyday life.

Milk Thistle/St Mary's Thistle (Silymarin/Silybum marinanum)

Milk Thistle or St Mary's Thistle, as it is commonly known, has been traditionally used as a liver tonic and liver protectant to support liver function and detoxification pathways. It also possesses antioxidative, anti-inflammatory and liver-regenerating properties as well as supporting immune function. Clinical studies prove it's beneficial role in supporting liver function and protecting against oxidative damage.

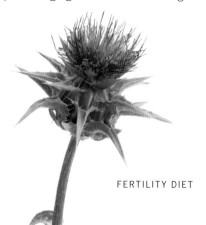

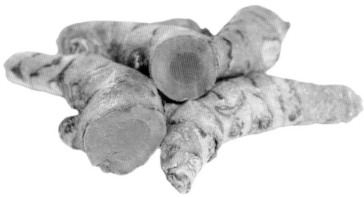

Turmeric

Turmeric supports detoxification pathways in the liver whilst also providing antioxidant and anti-inflammatory action, both of which can be beneficial to support fertility. Clinical studies have shown numerous biological activities particularly in reducing the impact of exposure to heavy metals including arsenic, cadmium, chromium, copper, lead and mercury on the liver, al of which can impact sperm quality and development. This can be especially beneficial for those previously or currently exposed to these toxins. The strong antioxidant action also protects liver cells against all forms of oxidative stress.

Reproductive function

Korean Ginseng (Panax ginseng)

Korean ginseng is one of the most widely used herbal medicines to support a range of reproductive concerns including fertility. It's use dates back over 2000 years. The broad-spectrum benefits of Korean ginseng for male health have established it as a premium male tonic. It has been shown to support testicular function, improve sperm health and survival rate as well as acting as an aphrodisiac. Korean ginseng also supports erectile response and has a strong history of success in improving erectile dysfunction. Korean ginseng also provides antioxidant activity as well as supporting

the stress response and energy production. Clinical studies show that supplementation with Panax ginseng results increased sperm count, improved motility, improvements in testosterone levels as well as significant improvement in general fertility parameters and testicular antioxidant activity.

Recommended dose – 1500 – 2000mg per day. Long term use is not suggested. If supplementing for longer than 1 month, it's recommended to use for 3 weeks in each month.

Tribulus

Has been traditionally and widely used to support male libido and sexual function. Recent clinical studies further support it's role in fertility showing positive improvements in sperm count and sperm motility as well as increasing testosterone levels.

Recommended dose – 1000 – 2000mg per day

Yohimbine (Pausinystalia yohimbe)

Yohimbine has been used as a pharmacological agent in the treatment of erectile dysfunction for over 70 years. Studies have shown that Yohimbine has a positive impact on overall male sexual performance as well as orgasmic dysfunction. Yohimbine has a long history of safe use, however its clinical activity is not limited to the reproductive organs and there have been some reports of headache, sweating and it may exacerbate hypertension, anxiety and sleeplessness. For this reason it is cautioned for those taking antidepressants or high blood pressure medication.

Recommended dose – 5.4mg 3 x per day

Withania somnifera/Indian ginseng

Withania is one of our oldest 'folk' medicines with use dating back to 6000BC. Withania has been traditionally used throughout the years as aphrodisiac and general tonic. Numerous clinical studies have supported this traditional therapeutic use as well as confirming its role in increasing sperm production and increasing serum testosterone levels. A recent placebo controlled trial showed significantly improved semen parameters with increased sperm count and improved sperm motility. Alongside these therapeutic benefits Withania also provides antioxidant activity and well as helping to reduce stress levels, which can greatly impact overall fertility. Psychological stress increases cortisol levels, which impacts sperm quality. Withania supplementation in stressed individuals has been shown to reduce cortisol levels leading to significant improvements in sperm count and motility.

Recommended dose – 3000mg – 9000mg per day

MACA root (Lepidium meyenii)

MACA has a long traditional use as a virility, libido and fertility tonic. It's believed to help promote sperm count and quality as well as supporting energy levels. Clinical studies have confirmed it's traditional use with subjects reporting increased sexual desire. One study also showed improvements in sperm count and quality. Although clinical data is fairly limited, this herbal 'superfood', makes useful addition to your therapeutic regime for its valuable nutrient profile of over 30 minerals and 60 plant nutrients.

Recommended dose – 1500 – 3000mg or 1 heaped tsp of MACA powder per day

Ginkgo Biloba

Ginkgo biloba has been traditionally used to support circulation as well as providing antioxidant activity. Thus, ginkgo is commonly prescribed for those suffering erectile dysfunction to help improve circulation to the reproductive organs. Clinical studies have largely focused on the use of Ginkgo in the treatment of antidepressant related erectile dysfunction, with a 76% success rate.

Recommended dose – 6000mg – 12,000mg per of dry leaf day

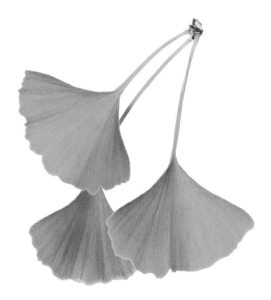

Diet

We are what we eat, and this relates to our offspring as well. Diet directly impacts sperm health. Research published by the American Society for Reproductive Medicine shows that a healthy diet including plenty of fish, vegetables and whole grains means better quality, more virile sperm. Poor diet, high in saturated and trans-fats means lower quality sperm and can impact sperm count. Although high protein diets have become popular amongst men for both weight loss and muscle gain, these should be used in moderation. Healthy protein levels are beneficial for both general health and fertility however excessive intake of meat and synthesised protein shakes and bars may negatively impact fertility. Diet should focus on whole foods as outlined below. For best results, men can also follow the 90 day fertility diet outlined in the book.

FOODS TO INCREASE
- ✓ Fresh vegetables, fruits
- ✓ Whole grains and legumes
- ✓ Nuts and seeds
- ✓ Fish
- ✓ Moderate intake of meat and dairy
- ✓ Eat organic where possible to avoid pesticides and herbicides
- ✓ Plenty of filtered or spring water

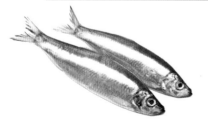

FOODS TO AVOID
- ✓ Processed foods as well as artificial sweeteners, additives and trans fats
- ✓ Fried and barbequed charcoal foods
- ✓ Food in plastic storage containers
- ✓ High intake of soy products

Exercise

Although there is no finite definition of exactly how many hours and how much intensity is optimal for each individual, most specialists agree that 45 minutes of activity, 5 times per week, is a great step towards boosting male fertility. Males are better able to cope with higher levels of intense exercise than females in relation to their fertility. So for those who already participate in more regular exercise than these recommended levels, that's likely to be fine, however it's not recommended to significantly increase your exercise load too suddenly. Maintenance or a gradual increase in exercise is ideal.

There is little evidence to suggest that one activity is more beneficial than another, however studies so suggest that frequent, long distance bike riding may have a negative impact on sperm production but increasing heat and reducing circulation to the testes. Although evidence is limited about the exact impact on fertility, it would be advisable to ensure you have a cushioned bike seat, avoid overly tight bike short and opt for breathable material and take regular breaks if participating in regular cycling.

When you're ready to start trying for a baby

SEX MATTERS

When to have sex

I'm often asked, "when and how often should we have sex when I'm trying to get pregnant?" The answer is a lot. There is a common misconception that it helps to 'save up' sperm until the precise moment to make sure the maximum amount of sperm are available to increase chances of one of them meeting the egg.

In reality, men produce millions of sperm every day, so there's no need to 'store up'. Of these millions, even with perfectly healthy sperm only a few thousand make it through the cervix into the fallopian tube to have a chance at meeting the egg. In fact too much 'older' stored sperm may actually get in the way of the fresh new sperm on their race to the egg. Also nature is not always precise, timing of ovulation varies from woman to woman and can even vary from month to month so knowing the exact moment

your egg begins its journey and is available for fertilization is difficult.

So having regular daily sex is absolutely fine, in fact it will improve your chances of conception. Some specialist recommend having sex daily or every second day throughout your cycle rather than timing your ovulation at all. This will improve chances of conception, but may also be tiring, stressful and can put a strain on relationships. It's important that sex not become a chore. Having regular, enjoyable sex is much more conducive to conception, than daily, stressful sex. Although female orgasm is not required for pregnancy to occur, the muscle contractions of orgasm can support the sperm on its journey to the uterus and extra natural lubrication can also smooth the path. It's also a great stress release! So if the idea of daily sex sounds exhausting, charting your cycles and becoming familiar with your fertile days enables you to increase sexual activity around these days in particular.

If natural lubrication becomes an issue it's important to choose a lubricant that will aid, rather than hinder, conception. Some lubricants contain spermicide, which kills sperm. Naturally these should not be used.

Make love as well as making baby

Ok yes, your ultimate aim right now is to have sex to make a baby. But sex isn't and shouldn't be just about baby making. Sex is an expression of love and intimacy. Don't forget this. It's easy to fall into a tedious 'sex on schedule' pattern, which can negatively impact your relationship and increase stress levels.

THESE USEFUL TIPS CAN HELP YOU BOTH ENJOY THE BABY MAKING PROCESS:
Talk
Set aside to talk openly and honestly about your feelings. Create an environment where you each feel comfortable discussing any anxieties or concerns so these can be addressed as a couple.

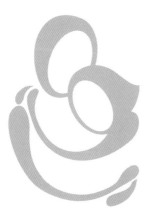

Nurture your relationship
It's easy to become so focused on bringing a new little being into your lives that you can forget to focus on you and what you mean to each other as a couple. Remind your partner how much they mean to you and how much you value them as a person, not just a baby making machine.

Be together
Take time to spend time together outside of the bedroom. Have a 'date night' or take regular walks together. Whatever you both enjoy doing as a couple.

Be intimate
Touching, kissing, cuddling, stroking, foreplay and experimentation. These things often go out the window when sex is seen simply as a means to an end. Enjoy some nights where you may not have sex at all, but simply enjoy feeling close to one another.

Can you have too much sex?

Simple answer is, no. Having more sex ensures that more sperm are available to fertilise the egg at ovulation. So light the candles, stock up on the chocolate and oysters and enjoy!

Do positions matter?

Again no. Healthy sperm are quick swimmers and are extremely adept at reaching their target once released, regardless of the sexual position.

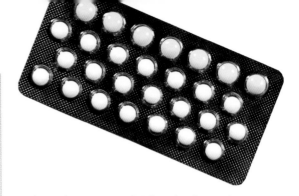

Going off the Pill

There are 2 main type of the Pill, the mini pill, which provides progesterone only and the more commonly used combined oral contraceptive (COC), which provides both progesterone and estrogen. There appears to be no significant difference in time to conception between either Pill or between the Pill and condom users.

Does it matter if I've been on the Pill for a long time?

Although some studies indicate a longer time to conception after long-term use of the Pill, this appears to be more related to advancing age, than the length of time the Pill has been used for. However, as discussed earlier, there is some evidence that long term use of the Pill may reduce uterine thickness and health of the uterine lining in some cases, which can reduce fertility.

How long until I'm fertile?

There's a common misconception that the Pill needs time to flush out of your system before you can conceive. In actual fact, the Pill is out of your system the very day after you stop taking it, that's why you need to take it every day at around the same time. Although it commonly takes a few months before ovulation begins normally again and on average it takes 4 – 8 months to fall pregnant.

However, although it is possible to conceive straight away after stopping the Pill, there are other reasons why you should wait.

The Pill can deplete the body of important nutrients including folate, B12 and B6 which are vital for DNA synthesis. When taking the Pill you are at greater risk of deficiency of these crucial nutrients, which leaves you at greater risk of miscarriage and birth defects. Deficiency of essential nutrients is associated with significant reproductive risks ranging from infertility to impaired fetal development and long term disease predisposition in the infant. For this reason you should begin boosting your intake of these essential nutrients through diet and supplementation even whilst taking the Pill so your levels are adequate when the time comes and ideally allow 3 – 4 months (remembering the 90 day life cycle of the egg) for your body to fully prepare for a healthy conception and pregnancy. See page 46 for the best nutritional supplement options.

"Perhaps strength doesn't reside in having never been broken, but in the courage required to grow strong in broken places."

~ Anonymous

Getting pregnant after IUD and other forms of contraception

Similar to the Pill, most forms of contraception use synthetic hormones, which can deplete the body of certain nutrients. Therefore I advise optimising your levels prior to stopping the contraception or taking other contraceptive measures for 3 – 4 months whilst you nourish your body in preparation for a healthy pregnancy.

IUD

There are 2 forms of IUD, a non-hormonal, copper implant and the newer progesterone releasing IUD (Mirena). There doesn't appear to be any significant difference in the time to conception between the 2 types of IUD, with studies showing on average 3 – 4 months to conceive. The main cause of infertility from IUD use is from scarring in the fallopian tubes stemming from chlamydia infection, which has shown to be higher in IUD users than other methods of birth control. However if you have been in a monogamous relationship, infection is unlikely.

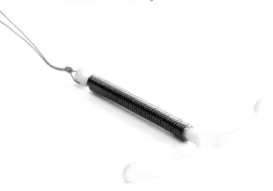

How long until I'm fertile?
Technically, you can conceive almost immediately after the IUD has been removed, but similar to the Pill, it can take a few months for ovulation to recommence.

Depo-Provera

Depo-Provera is an injection, which provides synthetic progesterone (medroxy-progesterone acetate) and is given every 3 months to prevent pregnancy. Once injections have ceased it can take anywhere between 2 months – 18 months for the progesterone metabolites to be no longer detectable in your system with an average time of 7 – 8 months.

How long until I'm fertile?
The time taken for ovulation to return, and conception to be possible, depends on how quickly the metabolites leave your system and can be anywhere from 3 months 18 months with an average time of 7 – 8 months.

Implanon

The Implanon is an implant around the sise of a matchstick, which is inserted into the inside of the upper arm. Similar to Depo-provera it releases synthetic progesterone. However the Implanon provides a different form of synthetic progesterone called etongestrel. Etongestrel is easier for the body to clear and is generally not detectable within 7 days of having the Implanon removed.

How long until I'm fertile?
A return of ovulation and fertility can occur within 3 months of having the Implanon removed.

Nuvaring

The Nuvaring is a small, flexible ring, which is inserted into the vagina. The contraceptive effects last for 3 weeks, during which time it slowly releases both synthetic estrogen and progesterone similar to those found in the Pill. The ring is then removed for 1 week during which time you'll have your period.

How long until I'm fertile?

The time taken for ovulation to return varies from around 2 weeks to just over a month with an average return of just under 3 weeks.

Ortho Evra Patch

The Patch is a relatively new form of contraception that provides both synthetic estrogen and progesterone through the skin and is applied weekly to prevent pregnancy. It can be worn on the upper outer arm, the upper torso front or back (excluding the breasts), stomach or buttock.

How long until I'm fertile?

Although no long-term studies have yet been done on the time to conception. Current studies show that is takes around 6 weeks for hormonal levels to revert back to normal.

HOW LONG UNTIL I'M PREGNANT?

Most women are at their fertile peak in their early to mid-20's. This gradually declines in the late 20's and then begins to rapidly decline after 35. In any given month, the average chance of conception for a women in early to mid-20's is around 25%, this declines to around 20% by the time you reach 30 and drops to only around 5% at the age of 40.

Most women under the age of 35 will fall pregnant within a year of trying. For women over 35 it can take longer than a year.

The up side is that there are many factors involved in conception and the progression of a successful pregnancy. So the answer to the question 'how long until I'm pregnant' will vary for everyone. However following the guidelines outlined in this book, will help improve your chances of conceiving sooner, no matter how old you are!

When to seek help

If you have been having unprotected sex for more than 12 months and you are under 35 years of age, this is when I would advised to seek professional help. For women over 35 it's recommended to seek help after you have been trying for 6 months.

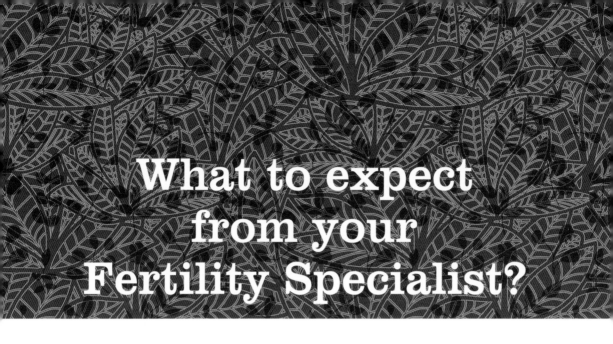

What to expect from your Fertility Specialist?

First of all, to visit a Medical Fertility Specialist you will need a referral from your GP. You should ideally request that the referral be for both you and your partner so you can both be treated if necessary.

Medical History

YOUR SPECIALIST WILL FIRST OF ALL NEED TO REVIEW YOUR MEDICAL HISTORY AS WELL AS YOUR PARTNERS, INCLUDING ISSUES SUCH AS:
✓ chronic illness
✓ prior surgeries
✓ medications
✓ birth control methods
✓ history of STD's
✓ have you ever been pregnant before
✓ are your periods regular
✓ any changes in your cycle
✓ Body Mass Index (BMI)
✓ exercise patterns
✓ caffeine, alcohol, tobacco or illegal
  drug use

Tests

Every couple is different and will present with their own set of unique circumstances. Therefore there is no ideal test, or set of tests for all couples. Outlined here are some of the tests your specialist may recommend depending on your particular presentation.

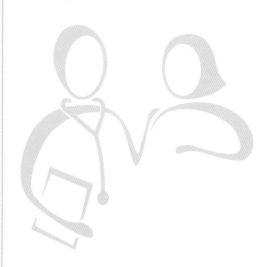

WOMEN

Basic testing

Depending on the level of testing your GP has already conducted your specialist will most likely organise some basic tests. These may include some or all of the following:

Pelvic examination
YOUR SPECIALIST WILL MOST LIKELY PERFORM A PELVIC EXAMINATION, THIS INVOLVES:

✓ lying on your back on an examination table with your abdomen exposed
✓ your specialist will manually feel your organs from the outside to assess size, shape and position
✓ you will then be asked to bend your knees or place your feet in stirrups
✓ a speculum is placed into the vagina to widen the opening and enable the cervix to be seen
✓ Pap smear may be performed at this time along with a sample of fluid to test for any potential infection
✓ A bimanual exam may also be performed where your specialist inserts two fingers into the vagina whilst using the other hand to feel above the area being felt inside to better assess the size and shape of your reproductive organs

General Pathology
✓ Rubella immunity (German measles)
✓ Hepatitis B and C immunity
✓ HIV check
✓ Full blood count to assess your blood group and thyroid status

Transvaginal Ultrasound
Unlike a regular ultrasound through the abdomen, a transvaginal ultrasound is performed by inserting an ultrasound wand into the vagina. Using this tool your specialist can view images of your cervix, uterus and ovaries and diagnose any abnormalities which may be affecting your fertility including cysts, fibroids and size of your ovaries. A transvaginal ultrasound may be performed in your specialist's rooms during your first or follow up appointments. It is also commonly used to confirm a pregnancy.

Ultrasound
Your specialist may request an ultrasound to assess the health of your reproductive organs. Ultrasounds are generally performed by an ultrasound specialists. Results are then sent back to your fertility specialist for review. An ultrasound is non-invasive and performed by running an ultrasound scanning machine over your abdomen to view your internal organs. An ultrasound allows your specialist to see any abnormalities such as fibroids, polyps and cysts as well as the size and health of your ovaries. Ultrasounds are also routinely performed to confirm healthy growth during pregnancy.

Progesterone level test
A progesterone level test is a blood test your specialist may request to confirm whether you are ovulating. As discussed earlier in this book, your progesterone levels rise after ovulation during your luteal phase, generally peaking between five to nine days after ovulation. Your specialist will generally

recommend having the blood test during this period, most commonly on day 21 if your cycle is a normal 26 – 30 days. If ovulation has not occurred, your progesterone levels will not be elevated. This indicates to your specialist that you are not ovulating. Another test will most likely be ordered to confirm the result the following month. If ovulation has occurred your blood test will show elevated progesterone levels. If the egg that has been release is not fertilised, your progesterone levels will drop back down again before the next menstrual cycle commences. If the egg has been fertilised then your progesterone levels will remain high (and congratulations you're pregnant!). This test is also commonly used when taking Clomid, to confirm that the medication is successfully stimulating ovulation.

Follicle stimulating hormone (FSH) test

As discussed on page 7 FSH helps regulate the menstrual cycle and the production of eggs in the ovaries. FSH levels are tested via a blood test generally performed on day three of the menstrual cycle. Your specialist may also request that the test be performed each day over several consecutive days to confirm your results. Your FSH levels will vary depending on the time of month the test is performed.

If your FHS levels are too low or too high, both these outcomes can impact your fertility. Low levels indicate poor egg production, which can impact ovulation. Low levels are commonly caused by high stress, starvation diets and low body weight. High levels indicate ovarian failure or that menopause has occurred. This test is also often performed to confirm the effectiveness of Clomid treatment. In this case the test will be performed before treatment on day 3 and again after treatment on day 10.

Other tests that may be recommended

Depending on the outcome of your medical history and basic testing, your specialist may recommend further tests to help diagnose the cause of your infertility.

Ovarian Reserve (AMH test)

This simple blood test measures Anti Mullerian Hormone (AMH). AMH is secreted by developing eggs within the ovaries. Levels of this hormone provide a good estimate of the number of eggs available in your ovaries, however it does not provide any information about the quality of your eggs. Your specialist will then compare your levels with the average for your age.

Sonohysterogram

This test involves an ultrasound as well as the insertion of a tiny tube into the cervix, which sends a dye into the uterus and fallopian tubes. This enables your specialist to determine if there are any blockages within your tubes.

"Fall seven times, get up eight."

~*Japanese proverb*

Hysterosalpingogram

This test uses x-ray to view the inside of the uterus and the fallopian tubes. A hysterosalpingogram helps determine whether there are any blockages in the fallopian tubes or any problems within the uterus, which may be preventing fertilization. This test is not as commonly performed due to the limited answers it provides in regards to ovarian and uterine health.

Laparoscopy

A laparoscopy is a more invasive test performed under general anaesthetic. This test is generally only performed if there are other indicators of reproductive issues such as suspected endometriosis or fibroids. One to 3 small incisions are made under the navel and above the above the pubic bone, through which a laparoscope (fibre optic telescope) is inserted. The exact location and number of incisions is generally based on your Specialists experience or your particular presentation. This enables your Specialist to view and assess the outside of your uterus, the ovaries, fallopian tubes and the pelvic cavity.

Laparoscopy may be performed purely for observation and diagnosis, or in some cases your Specialist may also provide treatment during the procedure, such as removal or reducing misplaced endometrial tissue or fibroids. Additional incisions may be required in this case.

Hysteroscopy

Unlike a laparoscopy, a hysteroscopy is performed to view the inside of the uterus, not the outside, and doesn't require incisions. A hysteroscope (fibre optic device similar to but smaller than a laparascope) is inserted through the cervix and into the uterus. This enables your Specialist to assess the size and shape of your uterus as well as the presence of scar tissue, fibroids or polyps. If abnormalities are found, your Specialist may treat these during the procedure, such as removing any small fibroids or polyps or helping to remove any blockages found in the opening of the fallopian tubes.

Anti-sperm antibody test

In rare cases, the women may develop an immune response to her partner's sperm, developing antibodies which attack, damage or kill sperm. An anti-sperm antibody test checks to see you are producing any of these antibodies.

Karyotype test

A karyotype test is a blood test, which examines the genetic material/chromosomes within cells to look for any problems that may be causing recurrent miscarriage or infertility.

Prolactin test

Prolactin is a hormone, which is high during pregnancy and breastfeeding to support milk production for the growing infant. Non-pregnant women and men also produce prolactin a low levels. Abnormally high levels in non-pregnant women can cause amenorrhea, nipple discharge and infertility. Your specialist may recommend a blood test to check your prolactin levels if you are having menstrual cycle issues or lack of ovulation.

MEN

Basic testing

Physical Examination

A physical examination of the testes is performed to check for the presence of any lumps, swelling, shrinking or any other signs of abnormality. Not all specialists will perform a physical examination for men

Semen analysis

A semen analysis is one of the first tests performed for males in couples having difficulty conceiving a child. Issues around sperm production, count and quality affect around one third of all couples experiencing infertility. The test is performed by ejaculating into a clean sample collection cup. This can either be done in a private room or bathroom within the clinic or if you live close to the testing centre you may be able to do the collection at home and then bring it to the clinic for testing. The main aim is that the sample be fresh. You will often be asked to abstain from sexual activity for 2 – 5 days prior to the test to help ensure sperm count is at its peak. However long periods of sexual inactivity can lead to less active sperm so it's ideal not to avoid sexual activity for more than 2 weeks prior to the test.

THE SAMPLE WILL BE TESTED FOR:

✓ Volume – the amount of sperm present in one ejaculation
✓ Sperm count – the number of sperm present in one ejaculation
✓ Sperm morphology – the percentage of sperm that are normal in shape
✓ Sperm motility – the percentage of sperm that are able to move in a normal forward direction
✓ Liquefaction time – the time taken for sperm to change from a thick gel consistency at the time of ejaculation to a liquid consistency. This normal occurs within 20 minutes.
✓ Ph – the acidity or alkalinity of the semen
✓ Fructose level – fructose is the form of sugar found in sperm to provide energy

Other tests that may be recommended

Depending on the outcome of the medical history and basic testing, your specialist may recommend further investigative testing

Testosterone levels

Testosterone levels are commonly checked especially if there are symptoms of erectile dysfunction, low sex drive or the result of the semen analysis showed low sperm count. Testosterone levels are checked via a blood test, which is often performed between 7 – 9am when testosterone levels are highest.

Prolactin test

Although largely known as a female hormone, men also produce low levels of prolactin. Higher than normal levels can lead to low sex drive, erectile dysfunction and infertility. Your specialist may recommend a blood test to check prolactin levels particularly if testosterone levels are low.

Testicular Ultrasound

An ultrasound may be performed on the testes to more accurately assess whether there are any issues within the testes, which may be affecting sperm.

Testicular Biopsy

A testicular biopsy is used to confirm whether there are sperm within the testes. It is very rare than males will produce no sperm, so this test is unlikely to be required unless there are other signs of lack of sperm production.

Karyotype test

A karyotype blood test may also be recommended for the male partner to assess the genetic material/chromosomes within cells for any issues that may be causing recurrent miscarriage or infertility.

CASE STUDY

- Susan, 29 years of age and Michael 29 years of age
- Trying to conceive for two and a half years
- 3 unsuccessful IVF attempts

Susan presented with endometriosis. A curette was performed in hopes to improve her fertility but when this wasn't successful they moved on to IVF. Susan and her husband Michael came to see me after 3 unsuccessful rounds of IVF with just one chemical pregnancy where the embryo implanted only to come away within a day. Their embryologist had suggested that her eggs were fragmented (i.e parts of the embryo's cells have broken away and are separated from the nucleus).

Alongside the diagnosed endometriosis and mild PMS, Susan also presented with low-grade asthma, immune issues, digestive discomfort with certain foods and she complained of always feeling fatigued and needing a nap.

A hair mineral analysis found high copper and slightly raised levels of mercury and aluminium as well as signs of poor adrenal function, electrolyte imbalance and low zinc. Other blood tests showed Vitamin D and iron were slightly low and she had borderline high fasting glucose levels.

Susan and Michael's diet had been based largely on carbohydrates, high sugary foods and low in vegetables and fruits.

I advised they stop trying to conceive for 4 months while health issues and nutritional deficiencies were addressed.

TREATMENT FOR BOTH SUSAN AND ANDREW INCLUDED:

✓ Three weeks of a gentle detox and eating a healthy eating plan including foods to specifically support liver function including eggs and green leafy vegetables
✓ Removing dairy and soy from Susan's diet, which were causing bowel disturbance
✓ Antioxidant and liver support herbs and nutrients
✓ Natural deodorant replaced Susan and Michael's regular antiperspirant to reduce the aluminium load
✓ Large high mercury fish such as tuna, barramundi, swordfish and flake were substituted with smaller fish like wild salmon and sardines

MICHAEL'S SPECIFIC TREATMENT INVOLVED:

✓ Stress management with adrenal support herbs
✓ Correction of low zinc levels through supplementation
✓ High potent B-complex and a broad spectrum antioxidant
✓ Fish oils for cellular health

SUSAN'S TREATMENT INVOLVED:

Diet modifications including:
✓ Wholefoods, low GI diet
✓ Cruciferous vegetables daily
✓ Avoiding dairy
✓ Limiting red meat.
✓ Vitamin C, vitamin E, lipoic acid and zinc supplementation to help reduce the egg fragmentation
✓ Fish oil to help improve the lipid outer layer of the eggs

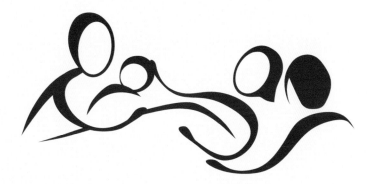

✓ Folate, vitamin B12 and B Complex
✓ Minerals based on her mineral deficiency
   profile

Just 5 weeks after her first visit Susan reported much better digestion and said her energy had doubled since first seeing me — she no longer needed her naps and was waking after 8 hours sleep and felt refreshed.

Susan and Michael were planning to go back to their IVF specialist after 4 months. This visit was not required as they conceived naturally after only three months.

Susan and Michael had a healthy boy, continued with their new healthy lifestyle and came back to see me when they wanted to try for baby number two, achieving another natural conception with a healthy baby girl. This previously infertile couple, have now just had their third child in another natural conception.

Written by Gina Fox, Naturopath and Fertility expert at Fertile Ground Health Group (www.fertileground.com.au). Gina is a leading fertility Naturopath in Melbourne, Australia.

"You're braver than you believe, and stronger than you seem, and smarter than you know."

~ Christopher Robin to Winnie the Pooh

90 day fertility diet

The 90 day fertility diet has been specifically designed to support egg health during the critical 90 day window as the immature follicle develops into the mature egg.

However, it's not just for the girls! This diet is also excellent for the male partner to support healthy sperm.

In general, the protein portion of a meal should be kept to around a palm size and vegetables, about 3 handfuls. However when following this diet, it's important to remember to tune into your body's hunger cues. Portions sizes may vary depending on your metabolism and desire for weight gain or weight loss.

Alterations that may be required for individual conditions are outlined below. Other than these individual changes, any alterations to the menus outlined should be minimal. The meals and snacks have been specifically planned to provide an ideal balance of important nutrients and should be followed for the full 90 days for maximum results.

Eating for weight loss

Even when aiming for weight loss, feeling hungry can lead to over eating and can actually slow the metabolism. The body recognises constant hunger signals as a sign that food is limited and can switch into starvation mode, conserving as much energy as possible. With today's abundance of food in our society, starvation is highly unlikely, however our body is programmed to see hunger and weight loss as a negative. Continued hunger and weight loss basically leads to death as far as our body is concerned, therefore weight gain is our body's aim (which is why it's easy for most of us to gain weight!). This is why starvation diets don't work and can just lead to rebound weight gain. For healthy weight loss you should consume portions, which lead to satiety but not over full. Remember that it takes around 20 minutes for the brain to recognise satiety cues from the stomach and give us a sense of being full. So always allow this time after a meal before deciding that you're still hungry.

Eating for weight gain

For weight gain, portion sizes should be generous and additional carbohydrates such as wholegrain bread can be included.

Eating for PCOS

The low GI nature of the 90 day fertility diet is excellent for those suffering PCOS.

Eating for Endometriosis

Wheat and gluten can aggravate symptoms of endometriosis and reduce your ability to conceive. The 90 day fertility diet is low in wheat and gluten, with the cleanse phase being completely wheat free. However, for those with endometriosis I would advise continuing to eat wheat and gluten free where possible by substituting either gluten free bread or substituting the bread based meals for a one of the bread free options. Dairy should also be limited and soy, almond, rice or other dairy free milk alternatives should be used instead.

Eating for Thyroid conditions and Uterine fibroids

The high fibre nature and wholefood base of the 90 day fertility diet makes it excellent for those suffering from thyroid conditions or fibroids.

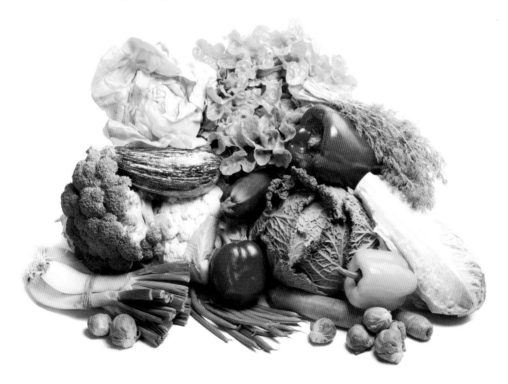

Week 1 - Cleanse	On waking	Breakfast	Snack
Monday	lemon juice in warm water	**Nourishing smoothie** + Prenatal multivitamin	Piece of fruit and handful of almonds or brazil nuts
Tuesday	lemon juice in warm water	**Morning refresh juice** + Prenatal multivitamin	Chai or other herbal tea plus handful of **superfood trail mix**
Wednesday	lemon juice in warm water	**Superfood Breakfast Smoothie** + Prenatal multivitamin	Carrot, celery and zucchini sticks with **avocado dip**
Thursday	lemon juice in warm water	**Berry and Avocado Smoothie** + Prenatal multivitamin	Piece of fruit and tub of natural yogurt
Friday	lemon juice in warm water	**Kale, pear and cucumber smoothie** + Prenatal multivitamin	Green tea with **antioxidant trail mix**
Saturday	lemon juice in warm water	**Superfood Breakfast Smoothie** + Prenatal multivitamin	Piece of fruit and handful of almonds or brazil nuts
Sunday	lemon juice in warm water	**Morning refresh juice** + Prenatal multivitamin	Chai or other herbal tea plus handful of **superfood trail mix**

Week 2 - Cleanse	On waking	Breakfast	Snack
Monday	lemon juice in warm water	**Morning refresh juice** + Prenatal multivitamin	Green tea with **antioxidant trail mix**
Tuesday	lemon juice in warm water	**Nourishing smoothie** + Prenatal multivitamin	Piece of fruit and handful of almonds or brazil nuts
Wednesday	lemon juice in warm water	**Morning refresh juice** + Prenatal multivitamin	Chai or other herbal tea plus handful of **superfood trail mix**
Thursday	lemon juice in warm water	**Kale, pear and cucumber smoothie** + Prenatal multivitamin	Piece of fruit and tub of natural yogurt
Friday	lemon juice in warm water	**Banana honey smoothie** + Prenatal multivitamin	Green tea and 2 **Protein balls**
Saturday	lemon juice in warm water	**Morning refresh juice** + Prenatal multivitamin	Carrot, celery and zucchini sticks with **avocado dip**
Sunday	lemon juice in warm water	**Chilled apple, cucumber and mint smoothie** + Prenatal multivitamin	Piece of fruit and tub of natural yogurt

Lunch	Snack	Dinner
Broccoli and almond soup with slice of gluten free bread if desired	Chai or other herbal tea plus handful of **superfood trail mix**	**Salmon with garlic asparagus and almonds.** Natural yoghurt with berries
Avocado and kiwi salad	**Chilled apple, cucumber and mint smoothie**	**Roast vegetable quinoa salad** with shredded chicken
Roast vegetable quinoa salad	Piece of fruit and handful of almonds or brazil nuts	**Pearl barley salad** with steamed rockling (or fish or your choice)
Pearl Barley Salad	**Kale, pear and cucumber smoothie**	**Ultimate veggie burger** with salad of tomato, beetroot, spinach and baby peas
Ultimate veggie burger with salad of rocket, cherry tomatoes and avocado	Green or chai tea and handful of almonds or brazil nuts	**Roast pumpkin curry and tahini yoghurt**
Spiced millet, cauliflower and pea burger with salad greens or vegetables	Piece of fruit and tub of natural yogurt	**Hearty salmon vegetable and noodle broth**
Hearty salmon vegetable and noodle broth	**Nourishing smoothie**	**Snapper with snow peas and toasted sesame seeds**

Lunch	Snack	Dinner
Roast vegetable quinoa salad	Piece of fruit and tub of natural yogurt	**Hearty salmon vegetable and noodle broth**
Hearty salmon vegetable and noodle broth	Chai or other herbal tea plus handful of **superfood trail mix**	**Roasted red pepper soup with mushroom and vegetable rice paper rolls**
mushroom and vegetable rice paper rolls	**Nourishing smoothie**	**Ultimate veggie burger** with salad of lettuce, tomato, avocado and mushrooms
Super greens soup with slice of gluten free bread if desired	Green tea with **antioxidant trail mix**	**Snapper with snow peas and toasted sesame seeds**
Avocado and kiwi salad	**Kale, pear and cucumber smoothie**	**Roast pumpkin curry and tahini yoghurt**
Roasted red pepper soup with slice of gluten free bread if desired	Piece of fruit and handful of almonds or brazil nuts	**Millet and cauliflower burgers with salad greens**
Millet and cauliflower burgers with salad greens	Chai or other herbal tea plus handful of **superfood trail mix**	**Sweet potato and green bean salad** with steamed rockling (or fish or your choice)

Week 3 - Cleanse	On waking	Breakfast	Snack
Monday	lemon juice in warm water	**Superfood Breakfast Smoothie** + Prenatal multivitamin	Green tea with **antioxidant trail mix**
Tuesday	lemon juice in warm water	**Nourishing smoothie** + Prenatal multivitamin	Carrot, celery and zucchini sticks with **avocado dip**
Wednesday	lemon juice in warm water	**Morning refresh juice** + Prenatal multivitamin	Piece of fruit and handful of almonds or brazil nuts
Thursday	lemon juice in warm water	**Banana honey smoothie** + Prenatal multivitamin	Chai or other herbal tea plus handful of **superfood trail mix**
Friday	lemon juice in warm water	**Superfood Breakfast Smoothie** + Prenatal multivitamin	Piece of fruit and tub of natural yogurt
Saturday	lemon juice in warm water	**Berry and Avocado Smoothie** + Prenatal multivitamin	Green tea with **antioxidant trail mix**
Sunday	lemon juice in warm water	**Nourishing smoothie** + Prenatal multivitamin	Piece of fruit and handful of almonds or brazil nuts
Week 4 - Nourish	**On waking**	**Breakfast**	**Snack**
Monday	lemon juice in warm water	**Banana and honey bruschetta** + prenatal multivitamin	Piece of fruit and tub of natural yogurt
Tuesday	lemon juice in warm water	Organic porrige topped with blueberries, sliced strawberries and chia seeds + prenatal multivitamin	Chai or other herbal tea plus handful of **superfood trail mix**
Wednesday	lemon juice in warm water	**Polenta Breakfast Muffin** + prenatal multivitamin	**Nourishing smoothie**
Thursday	lemon juice in warm water	Organic porrige topped with **Antioxidant trail mix** + prenatal multivitamin	Piece of fruit and handful of almonds or brazil nuts
Friday	lemon juice in warm water	Bircher museli + prenatal multivitamin	Green tea with **antioxidant trail mix**
Saturday	lemon juice in warm water	**Banana and honey bruschetta** + prenatal multivitamin	Piece of fruit and tub of natural yogurt
Sunday	lemon juice in warm water	Bircher museli + prenatal multivitamin	Carrot, celery and zucchini sticks with **avocado dip**

Lunch	Snack	Dinner
Sweet potato and green bean salad	Piece of fruit and tub of natural yogurt	**Super greens soup with mushroom and vegetable rice paper rolls**
Mushroom and vegetable rice paper rolls	Green tea with **antioxidant trail mix**	**Ultimate veggie burger** with salad of lettuce, tomato, avocado and mushrooms
Ultimate veggie burger with salad of rocket, cherry tomatoes and avocado	Carrot, celery and zucchini sticks with **hummus**	**Salmon with garlic asparagus and almonds.** Natural yoghurt with berries
Spiced millet, cauliflower and pea burger with salad greens or vegetables	Piece of fruit and handful of almonds or brazil nuts	**Hearty salmon vegetable and noodle broth**
Hearty salmon vegetable and noodle broth	Chai or other herbal tea plus handful of **superfood trail mix**	**Chickpea curry**
Chickpea curry	Carrot, celery and zucchini sticks with **honey roast carrot dip**	**Sweet potato and green bean salad** with steamed rockling (or fish or your choice)
Sweet potato and green bean salad	Chai or other herbal tea plus handful of superfood trail mix	**Snapper with snow peas and toasted sesame seeds**

Lunch	Snack	Dinner
Mushroom and vegetable rice paper rolls	Carrot, celery and zucchini sticks with **hummus**	**Sweet potato and green bean** salad with grilled chicken
Sweet potato and green bean salad	Piece of fruit and handful of almonds or brazil nuts	**Stir fry beef with asian greens**
Roasted vegetable barley salad	Green tea with **antioxidant trail mix**	Sweet potato and green bean salad with grilled salmon
Super greens soup with wholegrain bread	Piece of fruit and tub of natural yogurt	**Roast vegetable quinoa salad** with grilled fish of choice
Wholegrain sandwich with tinned salmon, rocket, tomato and avocacdo	**Berry and Avocado Smoothie**	**Steamed organic chicken breast in curry sauce**
Spiced millet, cauliflower and pea burger with salad greens or vegetables	Green tea with **antioxidant trail mix**	**Roasted brocolli and almond penne**
Tuna and cannelini bean open sandwich	Piece of fruit and handful of almonds or brazil nuts	**Roast pumpkin and spinach curry**

Week 5 - Nourish	On waking	Breakfast	Snack
Monday	lemon juice in warm water	Organic porrige topped with **Antioxidant trail mix** + prenatal multivitamin	Piece of fruit and handful of almonds or brazil nuts
Tuesday	lemon juice in warm water	**Banana and honey bruschetta** + prenatal multivitamin	**Berry and Avocado Smoothie**
Wednesday	lemon juice in warm water	Bircher museli + prenatal multivitamin	Piece of fruit and tub of natural yogurt
Thursday	lemon juice in warm water	Organic porrige topped with sliced strawberries, blueberries, and chia seeds + prenatal multivitamin	Carrot, celery and zucchini sticks with **honey roast carrot dip**
Friday	lemon juice in warm water	**Polenta Breakfast Muffin** + prenatal multivitamin	**Chilled apple, cucumber and mint smoothie**
Saturday	lemon juice in warm water	Bircher museli + prenatal multivitamin	Chai or other herbal tea plus handful of **superfood trail mix**
Sunday	lemon juice in warm water	Organic porrige topped with sliced banana and honey + prenatal multivitamin	Piece of fruit and handful of almonds or brazil nuts
Week 6 - Nourish	On waking	Breakfast	Snack
Monday	lemon juice in warm water	Bircher museli + prenatal multivitamin	Green tea with **antioxidant trail mix**
Tuesday	lemon juice in warm water	**Polenta Breakfast Muffin** + prenatal multivitamin	**Berry and Avocado Smoothie**
Wednesday	lemon juice in warm water	Organic porrige topped with **Antioxidant trail mix** + prenatal multivitamin	Carrot, celery and zucchini sticks with **avocado dip**
Thursday	lemon juice in warm water	Bircher museli + prenatal multivitamin	Piece of fruit and tub of natural yogurt
Friday	lemon juice in warm water	Organic porrige topped with sliced banana and honey + prenatal multivitamin	Carrot, celery and zucchini sticks with **avocado dip**
Saturday	lemon juice in warm water	**Polenta Breakfast Muffin** + prenatal multivitamin	Slice of date and seed loaf with honey spread
Sunday	lemon juice in warm water	Organic porrige topped with sliced banana and honey + prenatal multivitamin	**Nourishing smoothie**

Lunch	Snack	Dinner
Wholegrain or rye sandwich with cottage cheese, tomato, baby spinach, tasty cheese, grated carrot and avocado	Chai or other herbal tea plus handful of **superfood trail mix**	**Pearl Barley Salad** with grilled fish of choice
Pearl Barley Salad	Piece of fruit and tub of natural yogurt	**Roasted brocolli and almond penne**
Avocado and kiwi salad	Carrot, celery and zucchini sticks with **avocado dip**	Stir fry beef with asian greens
Broccoli and almond soup with slice of wholegrain toast	Green tea with **antioxidant trail mix**	**Ultimate chicken curry**
Wholegrain sandwich with boiled egg, spinach, tomato and avocacdo	**Banana honey smoothie**	**Chicken, pumpkin and bok choy noodle salad**
Chicken, pumpkin and bok choy noodle salad	**Kale, pear and cucumber smoothie** + Prenatal multivitamin	**Lamb apricot and date tagine**
Roasted red pepper soup with wholegrain or rye bread	**Slice of date and seed loaf** with honey spread	**Hearty salmon vegetable and noodle broth**

Lunch	Snack	Dinner
Hearty salmon vegetable and noodle broth	Chai or other herbal tea plus handful of **superfood trail mix**	**Chicken with quinoa mango and avocado salsa**
Mushroom and vegetable rice paper rolls	Piece of fruit and handful of almonds or brazil nuts	**Millet and cauliflower burgers with salad greens**
Roast vegetable quinoa salad	**Chilled apple, cucumber and mint smoothie**	**Roast pumpkin curry and tahini yoghurt**
Broccoli and almond soup with slice of wholegrain toast	Green tea with **antioxidant trail mix**	**Salmon with garlic asparagus and almonds.** Natural yoghurt with berries
Wholegrain or rye sandwich with cottage cheese, tomato, rocket, tasty cheese, grated carrot, cucumber and avocado	Piece of fruit and tub of natural yogurt	**Stir fry beef with asian greens**
Roasted vegetable barley salad	Carrot, celery and zucchini sticks with **honey roast carrot dip**	**Moroccan chicken quinoa**
Moroccan chicken quinoa	Piece of fruit and handful of almonds or brazil nuts	Lamb apricot and date tagine

Week 7 - Nourish	On waking	Breakfast	Snack
Monday	lemon juice in warm water	**Walnut and banana french toast** + prenatal multivitamin	Pea based protein shake
Tuesday	lemon juice in warm water	Organic porrige topped with **Antioxidant trail mix** + prenatal multivitamin	Green or herbal tea and 2 **protein balls**
Wednesday	lemon juice in warm water	Pea based protein shake with chia seeds and flaxseeds	Piece of fruit and tub of natural yogurt
Thursday	lemon juice in warm water	Bircher museli + prenatal multivitamin	Pea based protein shake
Friday	lemon juice in warm water	2 eggs omelette with tomatoes, spinach and parsely + prenatal multivitamin	**Kale, pear and cucumber smoothie**
Saturday	lemon juice in warm water	Pea based protein shake with chia seeds and flaxseeds + prenatal multivitamin	Tub of natural yogurt and handful of brazil nuts or almonds
Sunday	lemon juice in warm water	Poached eggs on wholegrain or rye toast + prenatal multivitamin	Green or herbal tea and **2 protein balls**

Week 8 - Strengthen	On waking	Breakfast	Snack
Monday	lemon juice in warm water	**Polenta Breakfast Muffin** + prenatal multivitamin	Green or herbal tea and 2 **protein balls**
Tuesday	lemon juice in warm water	2 egg omelette with tomatoes, spinach and parsely +prenatal multivitamin	Piece of fruit and handful of almonds or brazil nuts
Wednesday	lemon juice in warm water	Pea based protein shake with chia seeds and flaxseeds	**Chilled apple, cucumber and mint smoothie**
Thursday	lemon juice in warm water	Organic porrige topped with **Antioxidant trail mix** + prenatal multivitamin	Piece of fruit and tub of natural yogurt
Friday	lemon juice in warm water	2 poached eggs on wholegrain or rye toast + prenatal multivitamin	Green or herbal tea and 2 **protein balls**
Saturday	lemon juice in warm water	Bircher museli + prenatal multivitamin	Pea based protein shake
Sunday	lemon juice in warm water	**Walnut and banana french toast** + prenatal multivitamin	**Slice of date and seed loaf with honey spread**

Lunch	Snack	Dinner
Super greens soup with wholegrain bread	Carrot, celery and zucchini sticks with **hummus**	**Stir fry beef with asian greens**
Roast vegetable quinoa salad	**Banana honey smoothie**	**Salmon with garlic asparagus and almonds.** Natural yoghurt with berries
Tuna and cannelini bean open sandwich	Pea based protein shake	**Ultimate chicken curry**
Pearl Barley Salad	Carrot, celery and zucchini sticks with **avocado dip**	**Chicken, pumpkin and bok choy noodle salad**
Chicken, pumpkin and bok choy noodle salad	Piece of fruit and handful of almonds or brazil nuts	**Warm beef salad with cranberry dressing**
Broccoli and almond soup with slice of wholegrain toast	Green or herbal tea and 2 **protein balls**	**Moroccan chicken quinoa**
Wholegrain sandwich with cottage cheese, tomato, baby spinach, tasty cheese, grated carrot and avocado	**Slice of date and seed loaf with honey spread**	Lamb apricot and date tagine

Lunch	Snack	Dinner
Tuna and cannelini bean open sandwich	Chai or other herbal tea plus handful of **superfood trail mix**	**Salmon with garlic asparagus and almonds.** Natural yoghurt with berries
Wholegrain or rye sandwich with smoked salmon, capers, dill and cream cheese	Carrot, celery and zucchini sticks with **hummus**	**Ultimate veggie burger** or beef burger with salad of lettuce, tomato, avocado and feta
Roasted red pepper soup with wholegrain or rye bread	Green or herbal tea and 2 **protein balls**	**Stir fry beef with asian greens**
Wholegrain or rye sandwich with cottage cheese, tomato, rocket, tasty cheese, grated carrot, cucumber and avocado	Pea based protein shake	**Steamed organic chicken breast in curry sauce**
Mushroom and vegetable rice paper rolls	Green or herbal tea and 2 **protein balls**	Lean steak with steamed or grilled vegetables
Roast vegetable quinoa salad		**Snapper with snow peas and toasted sesame seeds**
Broccoli and almond soup with slice of wholegrain toast	Tub of natural yogurt and handful of brazil nuts or almonds	Chicken with quinoa mango and avocado salsa

Week 9 - Strengthen	On waking	Breakfast	Snack
Monday	lemon juice in warm water	Organic porrige topped with **Antioxidant trail mix** + prenatal multivitamin	Tub of natural yogurt and handful of brazil nuts or almonds
Tuesday	lemon juice in warm water	2 poached eggs on wholegrain or rye toast + prenatal multivitamin	Carrot, celery and zucchini sticks with **avocado dip**
Wednesday	lemon juice in warm water	Pea based protein shake with chia seeds and flaxseeds + prenatal multivitamin	Piece of fruit and handful of almonds or brazil nuts
Thursday	lemon juice in warm water	Bircher museli + prenatal multivitamin	Green or herbal tea and 2 **protein balls**
Friday	lemon juice in warm water	2 egg omelette with tomatoes, spinach and parsely + prenatal multivitamin	Chai or other herbal tea plus handful of **antioxidant trail mix**
Saturday	lemon juice in warm water	2 eggs scrambled on wholegrain or rye toast + prenatal multivitamin	Chai or other herbal tea plus handful of **superfood trail mix**
Sunday	lemon juice in warm water	Organic porrige topped with **Antioxidant trail mix** + prenatal multivitamin	**Nourishing smoothie**

Week 10 - Building and growth	On waking	Breakfast	Snack
Monday	lemon juice in warm water	**Walnut and banana french toast** + prenatal multivitamin	Green or herbal tea and 2 **protein balls**
Tuesday	lemon juice in warm water	2 eggs scrambled on wholegrain or rye toast + prenatal multivitamin	Piece of fruit and handful of almonds or brazil nuts
Wednesday	lemon juice in warm water	Bircher museli + prenatal multivitamin	**Berry and Avocado Smoothie**
Thursday	lemon juice in warm water	2 egg omelette with feta + prenatal multivitamin	Tub of natural yogurt and handful of brazil nuts or almonds
Friday	lemon juice in warm water	**Polenta Breakfast Muffin** + prenatal multivitamin	Green or herbal tea and 2 **protein balls**
Saturday	lemon juice in warm water	Organic porridge topped with **Antioxidant trail mix** + prenatal multivitamin	Chai or other herbal tea plus handful of **superfood trail mix**
Sunday	lemon juice in warm water	Pea based protein shake with chia seeds and flaxseeds + prenatal multivitamin	**Slice of date and seed loaf with honey spread**

Lunch	Snack	Dinner
Super greens soup with wholegrain bread	Chai or other herbal tea plus handful of **superfood trail mix**	**Sweet potato and green bean salad** with grilled salmon
Sweet potato and green bean salad	**Berry and Avocado Smoothie**	**Moroccan chicken quinoa**
Wholegrain or rye sandwich with smoked salmon, capers, dill and cream cheese	Green or herbal tea and 2 **protein balls**	**Stir fry beef with asian greens**
Pearl Barley Salad	Carrot, celery and zucchini sticks with **hummus**	**Lamb apricot and date tagine**
Tuna and cannelini bean open sandwich	Green or herbal tea and 2 **protein balls**	**Roasted brocolli and almond penne**
Avocado and kiwi salad	Carrot, celery and zucchini sticks with **avocado dip**	**Warm beef salad with cranberry dressing**
Warm beef salad with cranberry dressing	Piece of fruit and handful of almonds or brazil nuts	**Roast pumpkin and spinach curry**

Lunch	Snack	Dinner
Roasted red pepper soup with wholegrain or rye bread	Pea based protein shake	**Chicken, pumpkin and bok choy noodle salad**
Mushroom and vegetable rice paper rolls	Carrot, celery and zucchini sticks with **hummus**	Lean steak with steamed or grilled vegetables
Wholegrain sandwich with boiled egg, spinach, tomato and avocacdo	Chai or other herbal tea plus handful of **antioxidant trail mix**	**Pearl Barley Salad** with grilled fish of choice
Pearl Barley Salad	**Slice of date and seed loaf with honey spread**	**Ultimate chicken curry**
Wholegrain or rye sandwich with smoked salmon, capers, dill and cream cheese	**Nourishing smoothie**	**Salmon with garlic asparagus and almonds.** Natural yoghurt with berries
Tuna and cannelini bean open sandwich	Green or herbal tea and 2 **protein balls**	**Moroccan chicken quinoa**
Super greens soup with wholegrain bread	Carrot, celery and zucchini sticks with **avocado dip**	Lean steak with steamed or grilled vegetables

Week 11 - Building and growth	On waking	Breakfast	Snack
Monday	lemon juice in warm water	2 poached eggs on wholegrain or rye toast + prenatal multivitamin	**Morning refresh juice**
Tuesday	lemon juice in warm water	Bircher museli + prenatal multivitamin	Green or herbal tea and 2 **protein balls**
Wednesday	lemon juice in warm water	Pea based protein shake with chia seeds and flaxseeds + prenatal multivitamin	Chai or other herbal tea plus handful of **superfood trail mix**
Thursday	lemon juice in warm water	Organic porridge topped with **Antioxidant trail mix** + prenatal multivitamin	**Slice of date and seed loaf with honey spread**
Friday	lemon juice in warm water	Scrambled eggs on wholegrain or rye toast + prenatal multivitamin	Piece of fruit and handful of almonds or brazil nuts
Saturday	lemon juice in warm water	**Walnut and banana french toast** + prenatal multivitamin	**Nourishing smoothie**
Sunday	lemon juice in warm water	2 egg omelette with tomatoes, spinach and parsely + prenatal multivitamin	Chai or other herbal tea plus handful of **antioxidant trail mix**
Week 12 - Building and growth	On waking	Breakfast	Snack
Monday	lemon juice in warm water	**Polenta Breakfast Muffin** + prenatal multivitamin	Green or herbal tea and 2 **protein balls**
Tuesday	lemon juice in warm water	2 poached eggs on wholegrain or rye toast + prenatal multivitamin	**Morning refresh juice**
Wednesday	lemon juice in warm water	Organic porrige topped with **Antioxidant trail mix** + prenatal multivitamin	Tub of natural yogurt and handful of brazil nuts or almonds
Thursday	lemon juice in warm water	2 eggs scrambled on wholegrain or rye toast + prenatal multivitamin	Piece of fruit and handful of almonds or brazil nuts
Friday	lemon juice in warm water	Pea based protein shake with chia seeds and flaxseeds + prenatal multivitamin	Carrot, celery and zucchini sticks with **avocado dip**
Saturday	lemon juice in warm water	Bircher museli + prenatal multivitamin	Green or herbal tea and 2 **protein balls**
Sunday	lemon juice in warm water	2 egg omelette with spinach and feta + prenatal multivitamin	**Nourishing smoothie**

Lunch	Snack	Dinner
Moroccan chicken quinoa	Carrot, celery and zucchini sticks with **hummus**	**Lamb apricot and date tagine**
Wholegrain or rye sandwich with smoked salmon, capers, dill and cream cheese	Piece of fruit and handful of almonds or brazil nuts	**Chicken with quinoa mango and avocado salsa**
Super greens soup with wholegrain bread	Green or herbal tea and **2 protein balls**	Lean steak with steamed or grilled vegetables
Wholegrain sandwich with boiled egg, spinach, tomato and avocacdo	**Kale, pear and cucumber smoothie**	**Sweet potato and green bean salad** with steamed rockling (or fish or your choice)
Sweet potato and green bean salad	Carrot, celery and zucchini sticks with **avocado dip**	**Ultimate veggie burger** or beef burger with salad of lettuce, tomato, avocado and mushrooms
Tuna and cannelini bean open sandwich	Green or herbal tea and **2 protein balls**	**Hearty salmon vegetable and noodle broth**
Hearty salmon vegetable and noodle broth	Tub of natural yogurt and handful of brazil nuts or almonds	**Roast vegetable quinoa salad**

Lunch	Snack	Dinner
Wholegrain or rye sandwich with smoked salmon, capers, dill and cream cheese	Chai or other herbal tea plus handful of **antioxidant trail mix**	**Snapper with snow peas and sesame seeds**
Broccoli and almond soup with slice of wholegrain toast	Carrot, celery and zucchini sticks with **hummus**	**Chicken, pumpkin and bok choy noodle salad**
Chicken, pumpkin and bok choy noodle salad	Chai or other herbal tea plus handful of **superfood trail mix**	Lean steak with steamed or grilled vegetables
Tuna and cannelini bean open sandwich	**Kale, pear and cucumber smoothie**	**Millet and cauliflower burgers with salad greens**
Wholegrain sandwich with lettuce, tomato and avocacdo and shredded organic chicken and wholegrain mustard	**Slice of date and seed loaf with honey spread**	**Lamb apricot and date tagine**
Pearl Barley Salad	Pea based protein shake	**Salmon with garlic asparagus and almonds.** Natural yoghurt with berries
Avocado and kiwi salad	Tub of natural yogurt and handful of brazil nuts or almonds	**Warm beef salad with cranberry dressing**

Breakfast

Polenta breakfast muffins

Makes 12 muffins

Butter or oil for greasing

1¼ cups self-raising flour

2 tsp baking powder

1 tsp ground cumin

½ tsp ground coriander

Pink salt and freshly ground black pepper

¾ cup fine polenta

¼ cup grated parmesan

125g cherry tomatoes, halved

1 tsp freshly grated lemon zest

1 tbsp chopped fresh chives

1 tbsp chopped fresh parsley

2 eggs, lightly beaten

1 cup milk, soy milk or almond milk

2 tbsp lemon juice

1 tbsp olive oil

30g goat's cheese, crumbled

Preheat oven to 200°C. Grease twelve muffin pans with butter or oil. Sift flour, baking powder, cumin and coriander into a bowl. Season with pink salt and freshly ground black pepper.

Add polenta, parmesan, tomatoes, lemon zest, and chives to the flour mix. In a separate bowl, whisk eggs, milk, lemon juice and oil. Make a well in the dry ingredients, add egg mixture then stir until combined.

Divide between the twelve muffin pans. Top with goat's cheese. Bake for 20-30 minutes or until a skewer inserted into the centre comes out clean. Serve.

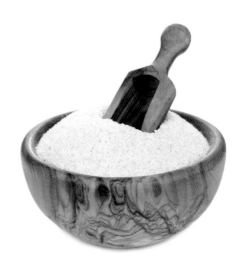

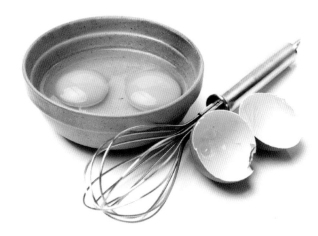

Walnut and banana french toast

Serves 4

1 small loaf wholegrain bread, unsliced

50g walnuts

1 banana, thinly sliced

2 free range organic eggs, lightly beaten

¼ cup organic milk, soy milk, almond or rice milk

1 tbsp butter

¼ cup honey or maple syrup

Cut the bread into thick slices. Use the tip of a sharp knife to cut small slits in the bread. Press the walnuts and banana slices into the holes. Whisk together the eggs and milk.

Melt the butter in a non-stick frypan. Gently dip the bread one slice at a time into the egg mixture until well coated. Cook the bread for 2 minutes each side or until golden brown. Place cooked slices on a plate and drizzle with honey or maple syrup.

Banana and honey bruschetta

2 slices of wholegrain bread

2 tbsp cottage cheese

1 small banana, sliced

1 tbsp honey

1 tbsp crushed walnuts

Toast the bread. Spread cottage cheese over the toast and top with sliced banana and drizzle with honey and crushed walnuts.

Smoothies

Morning refresh juice

1 apple, peeled and sliced

4 kale leaves, sliced

1 cup diced pineapple

1 cucumber, peeled and diced

½ cup fresh parsley, chopped

1 tbsp ginger, grated

Place all ingredients into a blender and process until smooth.

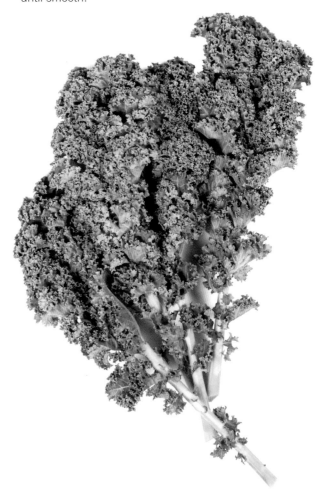

Chilled apple, cucumber and mint smoothie

1 small Lebanese cucumber, peeled and diced

¼ cup baby spinach or kale

1 apple, cored and sliced

½ cup lime juice

½ cup natural greek yoghurt

sprig of fresh mint, chopped

¼ cup coconut water

2 cups ice

Place all ingredients into a blender and process until smooth.

Kale, pear and cucumber smoothie

2 cups kale or baby spinach

1 ripe pear, chopped

2 dates, chopped

2 tbsp chopped coriander

1 lebanese cucumber, chopped

½ cup coconut water

Juice of 1 lemon

1 tsp turmeric

1 tbsp chia seeds or flaxseeds

Place all ingredients into a blender and process until smooth.

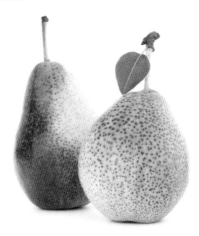

Berry and avocado smoothie

1 cup (125g) frozen berries
(blueberries, raspberries,
strawberries or combination)

½ ripe avocado, peeled
and diced

1½ cups (325ml) your
choice of milk

2 tsp honey

1 tbsp LSA mix

1 tbsp chia seeds

Place all ingredients into a blender and process
until smooth.

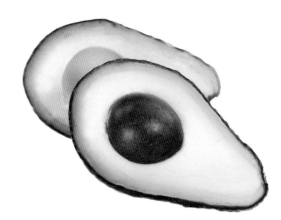

Nourishing smoothie

1 cup coconut water

1 cup oat milk

1 tbsp coconut oil

2 tsp flaxseed meal

2 tsp LSA mix

½ cup blueberries or
blackberries, or combination

2 tbsp natural yoghurt

pinch of cinnamon
to taste

tbsp of honey to sweeten
(optional)

Place all ingredients into a blender and blend
until smooth.

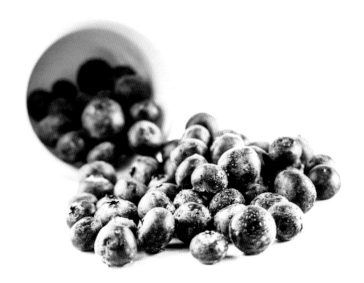

Superfood breakfast smoothie

½ cup organic rolled oats

½ cup blueberries
(or your choice of berries)

2 ripe bananas, peeled

1 cup your choice of milk

1 cup natural Greek
style yoghurt

2 tsp LSA

2 tsp chia seeds

2 tsp honey

Place all ingredients into a blender and process until smooth.

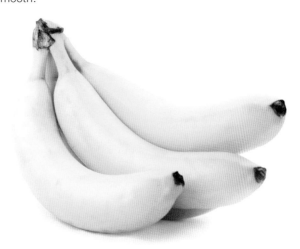

Banana honey smoothie

1 cup almond milk

½ cup natural yogurt

1 ripe banana

1 tbsp chia seeds

1 tbsp honey

Place all ingredients into a blender and process until smooth.

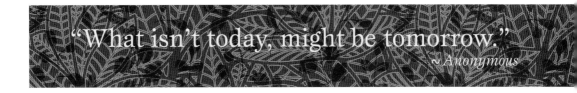

"What isn't today, might be tomorrow."
~ *Anonymous*

Soups

Super greens soup

Serves 4

1 broccoli, cut into florets

1 zucchini, diced into 1cm cubes

1 small bunch green asparagus, chopped into 2cm pieces

1 carrot, sliced

2 bok choy, roughly chopped

2 cloves of garlic, crushed or grated

2cm piece ginger, grated

4 shallots, coarsely diced

1 leek, sliced

2 stalks celery, sliced

500ml vegetable stock

3 bay leaves

tbsp parsley

sea salt and freshly cracked black pepper

Extra virgin olive oil and chopped sweet basil to serve

Heat a saucepan over medium heat, add garlic, shallots, leek and celery and sauté for about 1 minute.

Add remaining vegetables and herbs and sauté for about a minute then add vegetable stock. Bring to the boil then simmer for 15 minutes or until vegetables are tender.

Season with salt and pepper and remove bay leaves.

Set aside to cool then place soup in the blender and puree until smooth.

Serve with a sprinkle of extra virgin olive oil topped with pinch of chopped sweet basil.

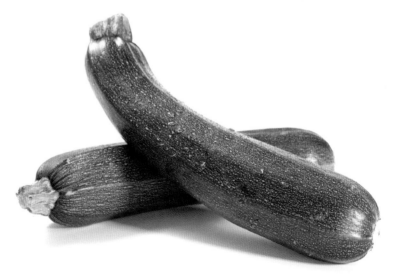

Broccoli and almond soup

Serves 4 - 6

750g broccoli florets

½ cup (50g) ground almonds

850ml vegetable stock

Sea salt and cracked black pepper

Place broccoli florets into a large saucepan, add the vegetable stock and bring to the boil. Simmer for 6 – 7 minutes until broccoli is tender. Add the ground almonds and blend with a handheld blender or food processor until smooth. Season to taste.

Roasted pepper soup

3 medium red peppers

4 tbsp olive oil

1 stalk celery, sliced

1 medium carrot, sliced

1 large leek, thinly sliced

1 tbsp fresh thyme, chopped

2 tbsp tomato paste

1 litre organic chicken or vegetable stock

1 small sweet potato, peeled and diced

Pink salt and freshly ground black pepper

Heat a saucepan over medium heat, add garlic, shallots, leek and celery and sauté for about 1 minute.

Add remaining vegetables and herbs and sauté for about a minute then add vegetable stock. Bring to the boil then simmer for 15 minutes or until vegetables are tender.

Season with salt and pepper and remove bay leaves.

Set aside to cool then place soup in the blender and puree until smooth.

Serve with a sprinkle of extra virgin olive oil topped with pinch of chopped sweet basil.

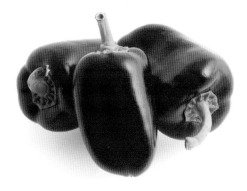

Lunches and dinners

Salmon with garlic asparagus and almonds

2 x salmon fillets,
skin on

1 tbsp parsley,
finely chopped

2 tbsp olive oil

2 small bunches
of asparagus

2 tbsp flaked almonds

1 garlic clove, crushed

chili flakes (optional)

Wedge of lemon

pink salt and freshly
ground black pepper

Preheat oven to 220 degrees Celsius.

Mix 1 tbsp olive oil with a pinch of pink salt and freshly
ground black pepper. Rub fillets with the oil mixture.
Place salmon fillets, skin side down, on a baking tray
and cook for 12 – 15 minutes or until meat is opaque
and flaky. Heat 1 tbsp oil in a pan over medium to high heat,
toss in the asparagus stalks and cook for around 30 seconds
or until golden. Add the garlic and chili flakes (if using).
Cook for a further minute or so until asparagus is just tender.
Sprinkle in the almond flakes and and parsley and toss
for 30 seconds or until almonds are golden. Divide the
asparagus between two plates and top with a salmon fillet.
Squeeze lemon over the dish and enjoy.

Note: *during pregnancy salmon
should always be eaten well cooked.*

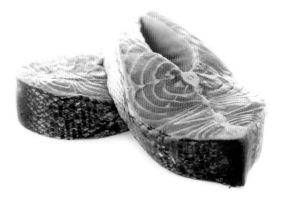

Avocado and kiwi salad

Serves 2

1 ripe avocado, diced

2 – 3 kiwi fruit, peeled
and diced

500g baby spinach

2 tbsp dried apricot diced

Cold pressed olive oil

Lemon juice

Place all ingredients in a large bowl and mix well
to combine. Drizzle with olive oil and lemon juice to taste.

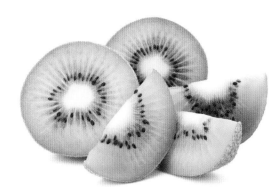

Moroccan chicken quinoa

Serves 2 - 4

2 chicken breasts

1.25 litres water or stock

1 cup quinoa

1 tsp ground cumin

1 tsp ground coriander

1 tbsp olive oil

Juice of 1 lemon

2 tbsp fresh coriander
leaves, chopped

1 tbsp fresh mint
leaves, chopped

3 tbsp raisins

pink salt and freshly
ground black pepper

Place chicken breasts in a saucepan with 750ml water
or stock (or enough cover breasts well). Bring to the boil
and simmer for around 15 minutes or until chicken
is cooked through. Remove chicken from saucepan
and set aside.

Place quinoa and remaining 500ml water or stock into
a saucepan, cover and bring to the boil then simmer
for 10 – 15 minutes or until water is absorbed. Fluff
quinoa with a fork and stir through remaining ingredients
adding salt and pepper to taste. Shred chicken breasts
and stir through quinoa mix. Serve with an extra sprinkling
of fresh coriander.

Chicken with quinoa, avocado and mango salsa

2 small organic free range chicken breasts

¾ cup quinoa

1 mango, diced into 1cm cubes

1 avocado, diced into 1cm cubes

Juice of one lemon

1 tsp chili flakes (optional)

Sea salt and freshly cracked pepper

Place quinoa in a saucepan, cover with 1½ cups seasoned water or stock. Bring to the boil and simmer covered for 12 minutes or until water is absorbed and quinoa is cooked. Chargrill chicken on a hot plate for 4 – 5 minutes each side or until cooked through. Set aside. Combine mango, avocado lemon juice and chili in a bowl, season with salt and pepper and stir lightly to combine. Place quinoa onto serving plates, slice chicken breasts and lay across quinoa, top with salsa mix and enjoy.

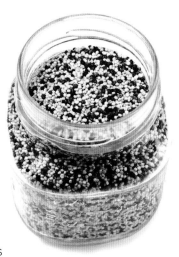

Roasted broccoli and almond penne

½ cup natural almonds

1 head broccoli, cut into florets

½ cup olive oil (place extra to for roasting)

1 cup fresh basil

2 cloves garlic, peeled

400g chopped tomatoes

pink salt and freshly ground black pepper

1 cup wholemeal penne pasta

Preheat oven to 180 degrees. Place almonds and broccoli separately on a baking tray, drizzle broccoli with olive oil. Roast until almonds for about 7 minutes or until golden. Continue to roast the broccoli for another 7 minutes or until tender. Transfer to a bowl and season with salt and pepper.

Bring a large pan of salted water to the boil. Place the pasta into the boiling water and cook for 10 minutes or as directed on the packet. While pasta is cooking pulse the almonds in a food processor until fine, add the garlic and process until finely chopped. Drizzle in ½ cup olive oil until blended then add basil and pulse until mixture forms a smooth paste. Poor mixture over the roasted broccoli and add chopped tomatoes. Season with salt and pepper as desired and stir through the pasta.

Sweet potato and green bean salad with sweet mustard dressing

SALAD

4 medium sweet potatoes, scrubbed and thinly sliced

1 tsp cinnamon

2 tbsp olive oil

pinch of pink salt

1 tsp thyme

250g green beans

¼ cup dried cranberries or acai berries or goji berries

¼ cup walnuts, lightly toasted and lightly crushed

150g baby spinach leaves

DRESSING

½ cup extra virgin olive oil

⅓ cup apple cider vinegar

1 tbsp maple syrup

1 tbsp mustard

pinch pink salt and freshly ground black pepper

Preheat oven to 180 degrees Celsius. Add the cinnamon, thyme and sea salt to the olive oil and toss through the sweet potato. Lay out on a baking tray and roast for 25 – 30 minutes or until potatoes and golden and tender.

Bring a saucepan of salted water to the boil, add the green beans and cook for 1 – 2 minutes or until beans are bright green. Remove and plunge straight into a bowl of ice water.

To prepare the dressing, combine vinegar, maple syrup, salt and pepper in a bowl. Whisk in olive oil and adjust seasoning to taste.

Combine beans, sweet potato, spinach leaves, cranberries and walnuts in a large salad bowl and toss through dressing.

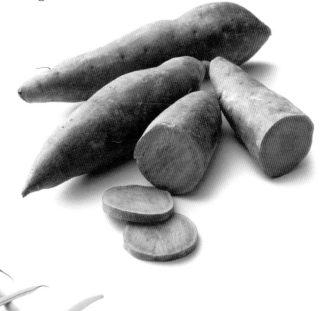

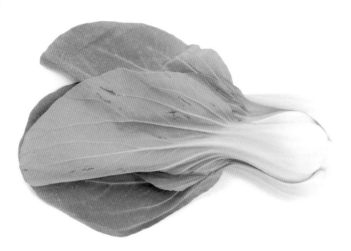

Chicken with quinoa, avocado and chicken pumpkin and bok choy noodle salad

Serves 6

150g egg noodles

1 bunch baby bok choy, roughly chopped

300g pumpkin, diced

Olive oil

¼ cup pine nuts

1 chicken breast

1 tbs salt-reduced soy sauce

2 tsp sesame oil

1 long red chili, thinly sliced

Preheat oven to 180 degrees Celsius. Lay diced pumpkin out on a tray, drizzle with olive oil and roast for 15 minutes. Add the pine nuts and roast for a further 5 minutes or until pine nuts are golden and pumpkin is soft and golden.

Bring a saucepan of seasoned water to a light boil, add the chicken breast and simmer for 15 minutes or until cooked through. Remove chicken and set aside to cool.

Refill saucepan with seasoned water and bring to the boil. Break noodles into quarters and add to boiling water, with bok choy.

Cook for 2 minutes. Drain.

Shred chicken breast with a fork and add to noodles and boy choy, then add the pumpkin, soy sauce and sesame oil. Gently toss until combined.

Spoon into bowls and serve topped with slices of chili.

Spiced chickpea curry

(Gluten free)

Makes 4 serves

2 tbsp coconut oil

2 tsp cumin seeds

1 brown onion, diced

2 garlic cloves, grated
or crushed

1 tsp fresh ginger grated

1 green chili, finely sliced

1 tsp garam masala

½ tsp turmeric

1 tsp ground coriander
seed

2 x 400g cans chickpeas,
rinsed and drained

2 x 400g cans diced
tomatoes

½ tsp pink salt

1 bunch coriander leaves,
roughly chopped

Heat oil in a large pan over a medium-high heat.
Add cumin seeds and cook until they pop. Add onion
and cook until softened but not brown. Add garlic,
ginger, chili and spices and cook, stirring, for 2 minutes.

Add chickpeas and stir to coat well with the spice mix.
Add tomatoes and salt, stir and bring to the boil.
Reduce heat, cover and simmer for 20-25 minutes,
stirring occasionally.

Serve with steamed brown or basmati rice or quinoa
and top with natural greek yoghurt mint leaves.

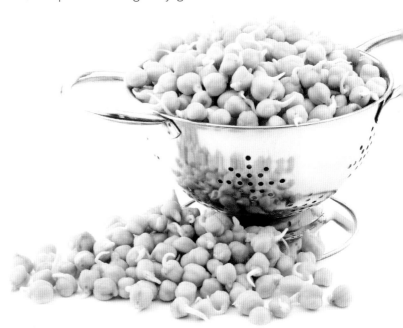

"There's no telling how many miles you
have to run while chasing a dream."

~ Anonymous

Tuna and cannellini bean open sandwich

Makes 4 serves

400g can cannellini
beans, drained and rinsed

300g good-quality tuna
in olive oil, drained and
flaked into large chunks

1 small red onion, finely sliced

10 cherry tomatoes, halved

large handful fresh
flat-leaf parsley leaves,
roughly chopped

100g fresh rocket

2 tbsp extra virgin olive oil

1 small lemon, juice

1 tsp wholegrain mustard

1 garlic clove, crushed

pink salt and freshly
ground black pepper

4 thick slices wholegrain
or rye bread

3 tbsp sun-dried tomato
paste

1 small lemon (extra),
cut into wedges, to serve

Combine cannellini beans, tuna, onion, tomato and parsley in a large bowl. In another bowl whisk the olive oil, lemon juice, mustard and garlic. Season with salt and pepper. Pour mustard mixture over bean mixture and toss to combine.

Top the bread with salad and serve garnished with fresh rocket.

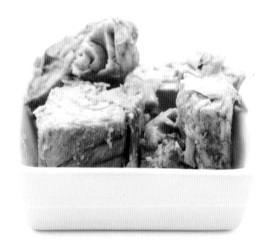

"Courage is going from failure to failure without losing enthusiasm."

~Winston Churchill

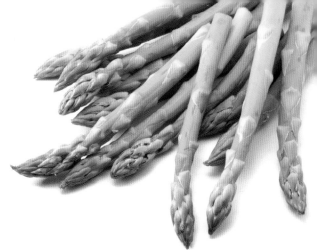

Warm beef salad
with cranberry dressing

Makes 4 serves

SALAD

½ tbsp coconut oil

1 small red onion,
cut into 8 slices

1 bunch asparagus,
trimmed and halved

4 x 150g lean beef
fillet steaks

Pink salt and freshly
ground black pepper

1 clove garlic, crushed

1 bunch watercress
sprigs, washed

DRESSING

½ cup cranberry
juice

2 tbsp red wine
vinegar

1 tbsp wholegrain
mustard

SALAD

Heat the oil in a large fry pan or wok over medium heat.
Add the onion and stir fry for 1 – 2 minutes until lightly
golden then remove and set aside.

Increase to medium-high heat, add asparagus and stir-fry
for 2 – 3 minutes or until bright green and just tender.
Set aside with the onion.

Season beef steaks with salt and pepper. Cook for about
4 minutes each side, or to your liking. Transfer to a plate,
cover with foil and set aside to rest for 5 minutes.

DRESSING

Add garlic to the pan, stirring for 1 minute or until fragrant
but not browned. Add the cranberry juice, bring to the boil
and cook uncovered for 4 minutes, stirring frequently, until
reduced by half. Remove from the heat, still in the vinegar
and mustard and season with salt and fresh cracked black
pepper to taste.

Slice steaks into thin slices. In a large bowl, combine beef,
onion, asparagus and watercress. Pour over dressing and
toss to combine. Serve immediately.

Poached organic chicken breast in curry sauce

Makes 4 serves

4 small organic free range chicken breast fillets

2 celery stalks and leaves, roughly chopped

1 bay leaf

pinch of pink salt

1 tbsp coconut oil

3 eschalots, peeled, diced

2 tbsp Thai green curry paste

400ml light coconut cream

1 tbsp fish sauce

1 tbsp lime juice

2 tsp grated palm or brown sugar

¼ cup mint leaves, plus extra to serve

¼ cup coriander leaves, plus extra to serve

Arrange chicken breasts around the base of a large saucepan and add enough water to cover well. Add the celery and bay leaf and season with pink salt. Bring to the boil and simmer for 10 minutes. Remove from heat and allow to cook through in liquid for a further 10 – 15 minutes or until chicken is cooked through. Remove chicken from poaching liquid and set aside on a large plate.

Heat oil in a frying pan over medium heat. Add eschalots and cook for 3 minutes or until softened but not browned. Add curry paste, stir and cook for 1 minute. Add coconut cream, fish sauce, lime juice and sugar. Stir until well combined and bring to the boil. Simmer for 2 minutes. Remove from heat and allow to cool. Pour mixture into a food processor. Add mint and coriander leaves and process until smooth. Return sauce to pan and reheat.

Sliced chicken diagonally and place onto plates. Spoon sauce over chicken and garnish with coriander and mint. Serve with quinoa, brown rice or salad greens.

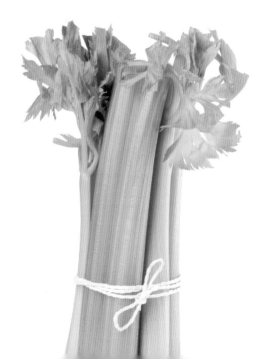

Nourishing salmon, vegetable and noodle broth

Makes 4 serves

1 tbsp coconut oil

3 cloves garlic

6 fine slices ginger

1 green chili, finely sliced

1 carrot, peeled
and thinly sliced

1 stalk celery, thinly sliced

3 spring onions, sliced
(plus extra to serve)

200g buckwheat soba
noodles

1 cup Chinese cabbage,
finely shredded

100g corn

100g snow peas

5 spring onions, diagonally
sliced

500g salmon fillets

2 tbsp sesame seeds,
lightly toasted

Heat oil in a large saucepan over low-medium heat.
Add the garlic, ginger and chili and cook for 3-4 minutes
until softened and but not browned. Add the carrot,
celery, spring onions and a litre of water. Bring to the boil.
Cover and simmer for about 20 minutes

Add the soba noodles and cook for 5 minutes or until
al dente. Add the cabbage, corn, snow peas and spring
onions and cook for 5 more minutes.

Chargrill the salmon in a pan until cooked to your liking.
Allow to cool slightly and break into bite-sized pieces
and stir through soup. Scatter with the sesame seeds
to serve.

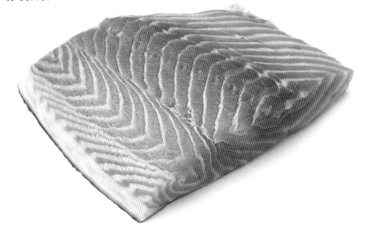

Mint and mushroom rice paper rolls

Makes 8

RICE PAPER ROLLS

80g dried fine egg or mung bean noodles

8 shiitake mushrooms

1 tbsp mirin

1 tbsp low-salt soy sauce or tamari

½ cup filtered water

8 x 22cm-diameter rice paper rounds

1 carrot, grated

100g snow peas, finely sliced

3 spring onions, finely sliced

1 tbsp fresh coriander leaves

1 tbsp fresh mint leaves

DIPPING SAUCE

2 tbsp lime juice

1 tbsp fish sauce

1 tbsp palm or raw sugar

½ large red chili, deseeded, finely diced

1 tbsp filtered water

Place noodles in a bowl. Cover with boiling water. Set aside for 5 minutes or until soft. Rinse and drain.

Place mushrooms in a saucepan, add mirin, soy sauce or tamari and water. Bring to boil. Reduce heat and simmer uncovered for 5 minutes. Set aside to cool. Remove mushrooms and reserve sauce. Remove and discard mushroom stalks. Thinly slice mushroom tops.

Soak one rice paper round in warm water until soft. Remove from water and top with a portion of noodles, mushrooms and each of the remaining ingredients. Drizzle with mushroom liquid. Fold at each end and roll to enclose. Repeat the above steps for each of the 8 rolls.

To make dipping sauce, combine ingredients and mix until well combined and sugar dissolves. Serve with rolls.

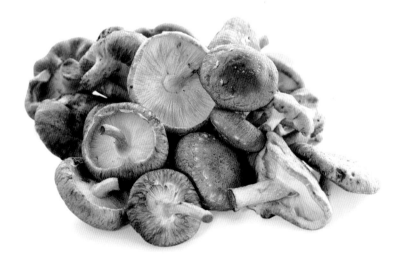

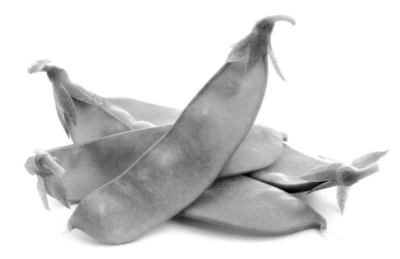

Snapper with snow peas and sesame seeds

Makes 4 serves

1 tbsp coconut or olive oil

4 fillets of snapper
(or other firm white fish)

1 small red onion,
finely sliced

1 large red capsicum,
deseeded, quartered
and finely sliced

2 zucchini, grated

60g snow peas,
finely sliced

¼ cup coriander,
chopped

2 tbsp extra-virgin
olive oil

Juice of 1 lemon

Freshly ground cracked
pepper and pink salt

2 tbsps sesame seeds,
toasted, to serve

Preheat oven to 200°C. Heat oil in a large frying pan over medium heat. Add fish fillets, skin-side up. Cook for 2 minutes or until browned underneath. Transfer to a plate and set aside

Place 4 x squares of baking paper, large enough to enclose each fillet, onto a flat surface. Place a fish fillet into the centre of each square.

Place onion, capsicum, zucchini, snow peas and coriander in a bowl. Add extra-virgin olive oil and toss until well combined.

Top each fillet with a portion of vegetable mix. Drizzle each fillet with lemon juice and season pink salt and black pepper.

Gather baking paper around fish fillets and secure with cooking string. Place parcels onto a baking tray. Bake in oven for 10-15 minutes or until fish is cooked through. Top with toasted sesame seeds and serve with salad greens.

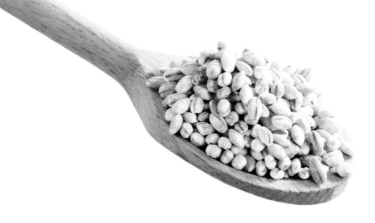

Roasted vegetable
barley salad

Serves 4 - 6

2 cups pearl barley

8 cloves garlic, unpeeled

1 red capsicum, cut
into slices

3 carrots, thickly sliced

2 red onions, cut
into 8 wedges

3 zucchini, thickly
sliced

2 tbsp extra virgin
olive oil

200g baby spinach
leaves

12 cherry tomatoes,
halved

¼ cup thai basil,
roughly chopped

Preheat oven to 180C.

Bring a saucepan of seasoned water to the boil, reduce
to a simmer, add the barley and simmer for 40 minutes
or until tender.

Place garlic, capsicum, carrot, onion and zucchini in
a large baking dish and drizzle with 1tbsp of the oil.
Roast for 30 - 40 minutes or until vegetables are tender
and golden. Squeeze garlic cloves from the shells
and set aside.

Place barley, roasted vegetables, spinach and basil
in a bowl and toss gently to combine.

Place garlic in a food processor with remaining tbsp
of olive oil. Blend until smooth, pour over salad mix
and toss well to combine. Serve.

Roast pumpkin and spinach curry

Makes 4 serves

1kg pumpkin, diced

2 tbsp cup peanut or olive oil

ground black pepper to taste

1 brown onion, diced

4 garlic cloves, grated or crushed

1 tsp ground coriander

1 tsp cumin

1 tsp chili powder

1 tsp turmeric

400g can diced tomatoes

1 litre low salt chicken stock

1 cup red lentils

400g can chickpeas, rinsed and drained

4 cups baby-spinach leaves, washed

Preheat oven to 200°C.

Place pumpkin on baking tray, drizzle with 1 tbsp oil and season with black pepper to taste.

Heat remaining oil in a large, deep frying pan over med-high heat. Add onions and garlic and cook, stirring, for 4-5 minutes until softened. Add coriander, cumin, chili powder, and turmeric and cook, stirring, for 1 minute until fragrant.

Add tomatoes, stock, and lentils. Bring to the boil and cook uncovered, stirring, for 15-20 minutes or until sauce thickens. Add chickpeas, spinach and roast pumpkin and cook until spinach wilts and chickpeas and pumpkin are warmed through. Serve with a dollop of natural greek yoghurt.

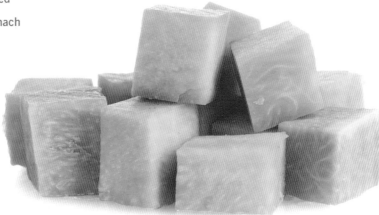

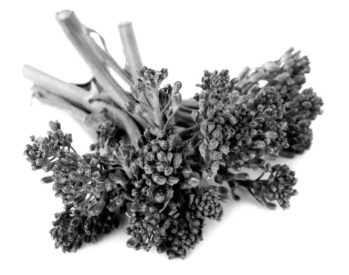

Stir fry beef with Asian greens

Makes 4 serves

2 tsp coconut oil

500g lean steak, thinly sliced

1 red onion, sliced

200g asparagus, sliced into 3 inch lengths

1 200g bunch broccolini, sliced into 3 inch lengths

1 200g bunch Chinese broccoli, roughly chopped

300g fresh rice noodles, cut into thick strips

⅓ cup fish sauce

2 tbsp oyster sauce

¼ grated palm or brown sugar

Freshly cracked black pepper to season

In a small bowl, whisk together the fish sauce, oyster sauce, sugar and cracked pepper and set aside.

Heat oil in a wok over high heat, add the beef and stir-fry until browned all over. Add the onion and stir-fry for 2-3 minutes. Add the asparagus, broccolini and Chinese broccoli and cook for 3 minutes or until becomes bright green.

Add the noodles to the wok and stir-fry for a further 5 minutes or until noodles and soft. Pour the sauce into the pan and stir well to coat noodles. Cook until sauce is heated through and serve immediately.

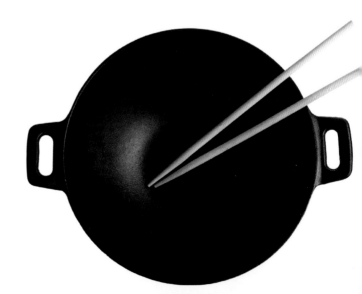

Millet, cauliflower, pea and ricotta fritters

⅓ cup hulled millet

300g cauliflower, cut into florets

1 cup frozen peas

2 eggs

½ cup fresh ricotta

⅓ cup milk

½ cup plain wholemeal or spelt flour

1 tsp ground cumin

1 tsp ground coriander

2 tsp finely grated lemon rind

2 tbsp chopped continental parsley

2 tbsp cup chopped coriander leaves

2 tbsp mint leaves

2 tbs olive oil

Heat a large saucepan over medium-high heat. Place millet in saucepan and stir for 1-2 minutes until fragrant. Add 1 cup of water, cover and bring to the boil. Reduce heat to low, and simmer for 20-25 minutes or until water is absorbed and millet is softened and cooked through. Remove from heat and leave to stand, covered, for 5 minutes. Fluff grains with a fork.

Meanwhile, steam or boil cauliflower for 6-7 minutes, adding peas in the last 2 minutes. Drain and remove cauliflower and peas and place in a large bowl. Roughly mash with a fork, then set aside and allow to cool. In another large bowl, whisk eggs, ricotta and milk, then gradually add flour, cumin and coriander. Stir in millet, cauliflower mixture, rind, parsley, mint and coriander.

Divide mixture into ¼ cup portions and roll into balls. Heat oil in frying pan over medium-high heat. Place balls in try pan, pressing down to flatten, and cook for about 3 minutes each side, or until golden. Serve topped with natural yoghurt and salad leaves or vegetables of your choice.

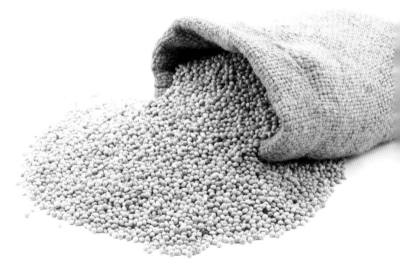

Lamb, apricot and date tagine

MARINADE

1 tbsp sweet paprika

2 tsp cumin

1 tbsp grated fresh ginger

¼ cayenne pepper

Freshly cracked black pepper to season

1 tsp olive oil

TAGINE

1.5kg lean, boneless lamb shoulder, cut into 2 inch cubes

1½ cups chicken or lamb stock

2 tomatoes, roughly grated

1 large onion, finely diced

4 garlic cloves, crushed or finely grated

Large pinch saffron threads

½ cup dried apricots, sliced

½ cup pitted dated, sliced

¼ cup, flaked almonds

⅓ cup coriander, roughly chopped

Combine paprika, cumin, ginger, cayenne, black pepper and olive oil in bowl. Add the lamb cubes and toss well to coat. Cover and place in the fridge to marinate for at least 1 hour ideally overnight.

Preheat oven to 180 degrees Celsius. Place the marinated lamb into casserole pot or tagine (approx. 10 cup capacity). Stir in the stock, tomatoes, onion, garlic and saffron. Replace the lid and bake covered for 2 ½ hours or until the lamb is almost tender. Stir in the apricots and dates and bake uncovered for a further 45 minutes or until sauce thickens and lamb is tender. Stir through the almonds and coriander and serve with cous cous or quinoa.

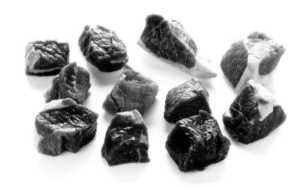

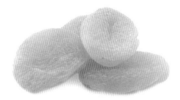

Ultimate chicken curry

1 tbsp coconut or olive oil

1kg organic free range chicken breast, cut into 1 inch chunks

1 brown onion, diced

3 garlic cloves, crushed or grated

3cm piece fresh ginger, grated

2 - 3 small red chilies, deseeded and finely chopped

1 tbsp ground coriander

2 tsp ground cumin

2 tsp curry powder

2 tsp pink salt

2 tsp paprika

400g can diced tomatoes

270ml can coconut milk

½ cup filtered water

6 cardamom pods, bruised

1 stalk lemongrass, trimmed and bruised

1 stalk fresh curry leaves or 4 dried curry leaves

¼ cup fresh coriander, chopped

Heat oil in a wok or large frying pan over a medium/high heat. Add the chicken and cook for 3 - 4 minutes or until browned all over. Set aside.

In the same pan add onion, garlic, ginger and chilies. Cook for 3 minutes or until soft but not browned. Add coriander, cumin, curry powder, salt and paprika. Stir until well combined. Cook for 1 minute. Add tomatoes, coconut milk and water to pan. Stir and bring to the boil. Return chicken to the pan with cardamom pods, lemongrass and curry leaves. Simmer uncovered for 25 minutes or until chicken is cooked through and sauce is slightly reduced.

Meanwhile, combine flours, cumin and chili. Season with salt and pepper. Stir in water until a thin batter forms. Half fill a medium saucepan with oil and place over a medium-high heat. When oil is hot, coat okra, 5-6 at a time, with batter and drop into hot oil. Cook for 2-3 minutes or until golden. Transfer to a wire rack covered with paper towel. Cook remaining okra. Serve curry with okra, papadums and coriander.

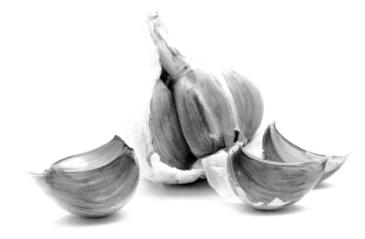

Snacks

Protein balls

40 dates

½ cup sunflower seeds

½ cup pumpkin seeks

1 cup desiccated coconut

5 tbsp pea based protein powder

1 tbsp coconut oil

2 tbsp almond butter or ABC butter

Soak dates in hot water for 5 minutes or until soft. In a food processor, place sunflower seeds, pumpkin seeks and ½ cup of the coconut and blend until well combined. Remove seed mixture into a bowl and set aside. Place the dates (drained), coconut oil and ABC butter into the food processor and blend until smooth. Pour the seed mixture back into the food processor along with the protein powder and blend until well combined. Roll into small balls then roll balls through remaining coconut to coat. Store in the fridge in an air tight container for up to 1 week.

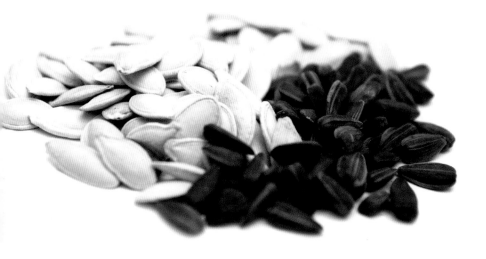

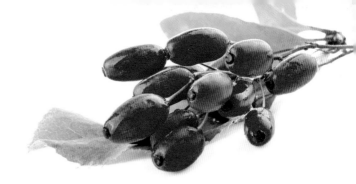

Superfood trail mix

½ cup natural almonds

½ cup pumpkin seeds

¼ cup sunflower seeds

½ cup natural sultanas

½ cup goji berries

¼ cup diced dried apricots

Combine all ingredients together and store in an airtight container.

Antioxidant trail mix

½ cup brazil nuts

½ cup pumpkin seeds

¼ cup sunflower seeds

½ cup goji berries

¼ cup diced dates

¼ cup diced dark chocolate

Combine all ingredients together and store in an airtight container.

"Even miracles take a little time"
~ Walt Disney

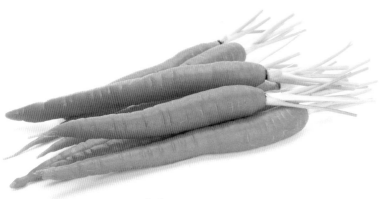

Honey roast carrot dip

5 carrots, peeled and
chopped into 3 cm pieces

2 tbsp cumin seeds

1 tbsp olive oil

Pink salt and freshly
ground black pepper

Preheat oven to 170 degree Celsius Combine all ingredients
and place on a baking tray. Roast for 20 – 30 minutes
or until soft and golden. Transfer to a food processor
and process until smooth.

Avocado dip

2 large avocados, diced

1 tomato, deseeded
and diced

1 garlic clove, crushed

2 tbsp lemon or lime juice

3 tsp chia seeds (optional)

drizzle with flaxseed oil
or good quality olive oil

Place avocado in a bowl and mash until almost smooth.
Add diced tomato, garlic, lemon or lime juice and chia seeds
if using. Stir well to combine. Drizzle with flaxseed oil
and serve with diced vegetables or wholewheat crackers.

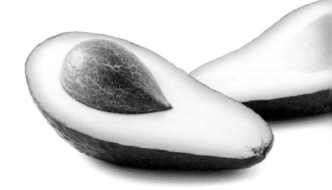

Date and seed loaf
with sesame and honey spread

LOAF

1½ cups pitted dates

1 cup filtered water

1 tsp bicarbonate
of soda

½ cup apple puree

2 tbsp olive or
coconut oil

1 cup organic plain
or spelt flour

1 egg, lightly beaten

1 tbsp sunflower
seeds + extra to top

1 tbsp chia seeds
+ extra to top

SPREAD

3 tbsp tahini

1 tbsp organic honey

Preheat oven to 180C. Grease and line a 10cm x 21cm loaf tin. In a saucepan, place dates and water. Cook over medium heat for 10 minutes until becomes a thick mixture. Remove from heat and stir in bicarbonate of soda. Transfer to a bowl and allow to cool slightly. Fold through the apple puree, oil, flour, egg and sunflower seeds. Spoon into prepared tin, sprinkle with the extra sunflower and chia seeds and bake in preheated oven for 30-40 minutes or until a skewer comes out clean when inserted in the centre. For the spread, mix the tahini and honey in a bowl. When cooled, sliced the loaf and serve with the honey spread.

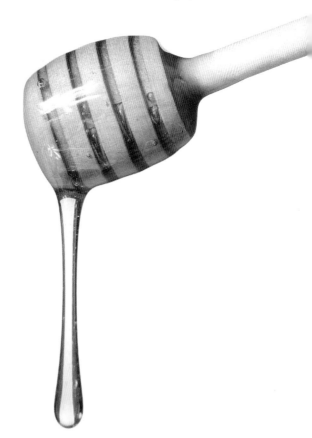

Index